613

AUG - 7 2001

YOUNG AT ANY AGE

A Book of Lists

Prescriptions for Longevity: Sense and Science

Pointers for a Healthy 100 Years

Abdullah Fatteh, M.D., Ph.D., LL.B.

Naaz Fatteh, M.D.

BROOKLINE BOOKS, CAMBRIDGE, MA

Copyright © 2001 by Abdullah Fatteh and Naaz Fatteh

All rights reserved. No part of this publication may be reproduced or transmitted in any form or by any means, mechanical or electronic, including photocopying, recording or any other information storage or retrieval system, without the written permission of the authors.

Library of Congress Cataloging-in-Publication Data

Fatteh, Abdullah.
Young at Any Age: prescriptions for longevity: sense and science pointers for a healthy 100 years: a book of lists/ by Abdullah Fatteh, Naaz Fatteh.
p. cm.
Includes bibliography and references and index.
ISBN 1-57129-083-4
1. Longevity. 2. Aging. 3. Self-care, Health I. Fatteh, Naaz. II. Title
RA776.75.F38 2000
613-dc21   00-010710
                                                                                           CIP
Published in the USA by Bang Printing
10 9 8 7 6 5 4 3 2 1

Notice to Readers

This book is intended as a reference document. The information included here is designed to provide general guidance for your health and longevity. It should not be construed as a substitute for any specific treatments prescribed for you by your physician. To determine what is appropriate for you, you are advised to consult your doctor. The authors and the publisher expressly disclaim responsibility for any adverse effects resulting from the use of information presented in this book.

Published by
Brookline Books
P.O. Box 381047 • Cambridge, MA 02238-1047
Order toll-free: 1-800-666-BOOK

In Fond Memory of

Our Parents

and

Mahatma Gandhi
John F. Kennedy
Martin Luther King, Jr.

*three giants whose lives were
shortened by bullets leaving the world poorer.*

613 F254y

Fatteh, Abdullah.

Young at any age

Contents

Authors' Preface xiii
From the Senior Author xiv
Acknowledgments xvi

PART I.
Focus on Facts

SECTION I. Perspectives on Longevity

1   Introduction 5

2   Primary Prescriptions:
     Ten Health Commandments 11

3   Ten Storytellers in Their Nineties: Their Gold
     Standards and Prescriptions for Longevity 13

SECTION II. The Critical Role of Diet

4   Foods for Longevity: Things You Must Know 25

5   Ten Famous Diets:
     Objective Analysis and Advice 42

6   International Restaurants:
     How to Eat Healthy at Each 59

7 Ten Fast Foods: Yes, They Are OK 74
8 Food as Medicine: Diet Prescriptions 83

SECTION III. Magic Bullets

9 Who Says There Are No Magic Bullets?
   Eight Of Them Are Right Here 103
10 Ten Other "Magic Bullets"
   Some Good, Some Bad, Some Ugly 125

SECTION IV. Exercise

11 Exercise: The Ten Best Ways 145
12 Stretching 148
13 Walking 158
14 Running, Safely 162
15 Bicycling for One Hundred Years 164
16 Water Exercises 171

SECTION V. Life Style Changes and Longevity

17 Smoking 193
18 Ten Best Ideas For Weight Control 198
19 Stress Busting Strategies 207

20 The Power Of Sleep 214
21 Love 222

SECTION VI. Caring for Your Body: A Systemic Approach to Longevity

22 Caring for Your Body: The Major Systems.................227
23 Action Plans for Each of the Ten Decades 249
24 Beating the Major Killers 257
    I.   Heart Disease: The Common Killer, Prevent It...............257
    II. Conquer the AIDS Virus..258
    III. Accidents Kill, Stop Them...259
    IV. Improve the Odds Against Cancer..............................260
    V. Obesity is a Disease, Trim It...262
    VI. Hypertension: The Silent Killer, Control It.....................263
    VII. Do Yourself and Others a Favor: Don't Light Up...........264
    VIII. Suicides: Prevent Them...264
    IX. Murder Mania: Cure It..265
    X. Influenza and Pneumonia: Don't Wait, Vaccinate............265

PART II.
Prescriptions for Longevity: The Best Practices

25 100 Prescriptions to Live to Be 100 271
    I.   Caring for Your Body...271
    II. Ten General Medical Prescriptions..............................278
    III. Some Diet Prescriptions..287

IV.	Exercise Prescriptions	295
V.	Prescriptions for Reducing Stress	303
VI.	Prescriptions for Weight Control	311
VII.	Social, Emotional Prescriptions	320
VIII.	Mental – Spiritual Prescriptions	329
IX.	Good General Prescriptions	338
X.	Ten Simply Best Prescriptions	345

Appendix A 357
Appendix B 359

TABLES

Table 1.1	Life Expectancies Worldwide	7
Table 1.2	Life Expectancy at 65, United States	8
Table 4.1	Daily Protein Requirement	26
Table 4.2	Ten Good & Bad Oils	29
Table 4.3	Cholesterol in Commonly Used Foods	31
Table 4.4	Ten Best Fruits	32
Table 4.5	Ten Best Vegetables	34
Table 4.6	Ten Best Grains	35
Table 5.1	Step I Diet Daily Intake	45
Table 5.2	Maximum Saturated Fat Intake	46
Table 8.1	The Nutritional Value of Ten Common Drinks	95
Table 8.2	Ten Best Sources of Fiber	98
Table 9.1	Ten Best Sources of Vitamin A	105
Table 9.2	Ten Best Sources of Vitamin C	106
Table 9.3	Ten Best Sources of Vitamin E	109
Table 9.4	Ten Best Sources of Calcium	115
Table 9.5	Calcium: Recommended Daily Requirement	116
Table 9.6	Ten Best Sources of Folate	118
Table 9.7	Folates: Recommended Daily Requirement	119

Table 9.8	Best Sources of Zinc	120
Table 9.9	Ten Best Sources of Minerals	121
Table 9.10	Ten Best Sources of Vitamin B12	122
Table 11.1	Energy Expenditure for 160 lb Person	146
Table 18.1	Desired Weight Daily Calorie Maintenance	199
Table 18.2	BMI: Degree of Risk & Treatment Options	201
Table 18.3	Side Effects of Popular Diet Medications	205
Table 19.1	Stress Level of Major Life Events	208
Table 20.1	Necessary Sleep Levels	215
Table 20.2	Caffeine Content in Beverages	217
Table 22.1	Ten Most Common Causes of Death Globally	228
Table 22.2	Percentage of People Over 65 with Common Chronic Conditions	229
Table 22.3	Ten Best Sources of Iron	232
Table 25.1	Top Ten Complaints of People Using Over-the-Counter Drugs	281
Table 25.2	Calories in Alcohol	291
Table 25.3	Calories in Soda	317
Table A.1	Recommended Childhood Immunization Schedule, United States, Jan.-Dec. 1998	357
Table A.2	Body Mass Index	358
Table B.1	Vitamins: Symptoms and Signs of Deficiency and Overdose	359
Table B.2	Minerals: Symptoms and Signs of Deficiency and Overdose	361

DIAGRAMS

Diagram 1	Food Pyramid	44
Diagram 2-13	Stretching Exercises Illustrated	155-157
Diagram 14-33	Water Exercises Illustrated	184-189

Authors' Preface

This book is about living longer and healthier. It is for all ages. It has ten merits:

1. It is a book of lists.
2. It contains the ten best of everything to increase longevity.
3. It is simple. It is as easy to read as counting from one to ten. No medical jargon.
4. It contains the latest scientifically sound medical information to achieve a longer, healthier life. It contains pearls of wisdom picked from our brains, clinical experience and from every available book dealing directly and indirectly with the subject of longevity.
5. It represents the collective wisdom of the medical establishment. It presents no controversial information or recommendations.
6. It creates a perfect marriage of common sense and science.
7. It covers every aspect of your lifestyle, including the right foods (with many healthy recipes), and exercises for all ages (illustrated by diagrams).
8. It presents totally unbiased conclusions and counsel on everything affecting longevity.
9. If you are in your nineties it tells you what, how and why.
10. It is an *encyclopedia of prescriptions* to make you feel better, look younger, function better and live longer. It is indeed a book for anyone who wants simple, reliable, useful and practical information.

Abdullah Fatteh, M.D., Ph.D., LL.B.
Naaz Fatteh, M.D.

From the Senior Author

"I shall die young, at whatever age the experience occurs."

– Ruth Bernard

I practice what I preach. So, as the senior author, first let me tell you what I do. Then, I will tell you what you should do. Let me start with a few facts of my life for proper perspective.

I was born in a remote village in India, population 600, where there were no doctors. My father, a farmer, businessman, Islamic priest and a novelist died at the age of 63 from chronic lung disease. My mother died from pneumonia at 42. My eldest brother died at 60 from a stroke, next eldest at 55 from a heart attack, another brother at 51 from a heart attack and one brother died at the age of 34 from a heart attack.

I have worked hard all my life. After getting medical and law degrees and a Ph.D. in Pathology, I taught in medical schools. I simultaneously worked as a Medical Examiner in several county, state and federal governments for 20 years and have performed over 7,000 autopsies. For the last 20 years, I have been working full-time as a family physician and part-time as a pathologist. To stay mentally active, I write. This is my sixth book. In addition, I have published more than 60 articles in scientific journals or books and numerous other publications in the non-medical press.

I eat three meals a day with no snacks between meals. I eat everything but keep the total calorie intake from fat at about 25%. I drink one or two alcoholic drinks before dinner most days and never touch soft drinks. I drink over eight glasses of water daily. I walk four miles at a fast pace, six days a week. My other important hobby is playing with my grandchildren who keep me physically active. They give me a fun workout every day. I am 5'9" and have maintained my weight at about 144 pounds for the last 40 years.

At the age of eight I was on a deathbed. A smallpox epidemic had afflicted almost everyone in the village. We had no doctor. My father summoned a physician practicing in a neighboring town. Seeing my whole body covered with smallpox lesions the doctor uttered: "He won't make it, let him go peacefully." The epidemic killed one-third of the village population. Against all odds I was a lucky survivor. At age 66 I was hit with chicken pox. On December 31, 1999, with open heart surgery, I received five coronary artery bypass grafts.

I have been married for 40 years. I have a lot of positive stress, very little negative stress. I pray every day. My latest total cholesterol is 174; triglycerides 81, my good cholesterol (HDL) is 47 and the bad cholesterol (LDL) 108. The genetic risk has run heavily against me, but with a good lifestyle I have come out a survivor. I am young and refuse to get old. Sixty-one percent of Americans say they want to live to be 100 or older. I do, too.

I am healthy, but I face disturbing questions every day from within. Why did my relatives have to die so early? What can I do to help others? One part of my mission in life was to educate my children. Now, they are all physicians, helping others. The youngest one, the co-author of this book, made a commitment to help me complete the second part of the mission: *to create prescriptions that will help all fellow human beings live healthier and longer.* Our path has included the review of over 400 books and almost all the current scientific literature on the subject of longevity. Combining our experiences and our knowledge derived from education and research, we have crystallized all these prescriptions for you. You will find in this book facts about everything you need to know to live to be 100 or more.

Abdullah Fatteh, M.D., Ph.D., LL.B.

Acknowledgments

In the preparation of all the prescriptions presented in this book we owe a great deal of indebtedness.

First, our family members provided an unflinching support. Sabiha Khan, M.D., our partner in medical practice, was always considerate and generous in letting us get out of the office to research and write this book. She also contributed in various ways by providing advice, encouragement and ideas. We can not thank her enough. Faiz Fatteh, M.D., Shahnaz Fatteh, M.D. and Mohammed Khan, M.D. individually and jointly contributed immensely with their youthful wisdom, knowledge of recent advances in medicine, and constructive criticism. This book is the brain child of all six physicians in our family.

Mahlaqua Fatteh, wife and mother, was a silent but major contributor in her own way. She is the best cook we know and always came up with great ideas for healthy menus. Our love and thankfulness is extended to her.

We are also deeply grateful to the ten story tellers for their messages. In the preparation of the book the help of Sareh Beladi, Kathy Bushouse, Caren Neile, Vicki Short, J.D. and Brittany Wallman is deeply appreciated.

Our associate, Cenk Sengun, M.D., prepared all the illustrations. We thank him for his patience and care.

We thank Felisa Sarabando-Gomez and Lisa Vrooman for being so meticulous in typing this book.

Finally, we extend our sincere thanks to our publisher, Milt Budoff, who made the production of this book a real pleasure.

Abdullah Fatteh, M.D., Ph.D., LL.B.
Naaz Fatteh, M.D.

PART I
Focus on Facts

Section I.

Perspectives on Longevity

Chapter 1

Introduction

Fundamental Beliefs

Let us start with *ten fundamental beliefs* you must have to qualify to read this book:

1. Every individual in each decade of life can contribute to the process of living longer.
2. The best way to slow aging is to start working on it early in life and continue through every decade of life.
3. Aging, to a large extent, is a result of many self-inflicted insults on the body; the insults created by a lifestyle of excess eating, lapses in conditioning of the body through lack of physical activity, and exposure to unwanted, unnecessary elements.
4. Aging invites early death; anti-aging attitude and efforts delay it.
5. Death is inevitable but aging can be slowed.
6. The metabolic changes, decreased activity levels, increased vulnerability to degenerative diseases, free radical attacks and the weakening of the immune system contribute to aging.
7. The aging process accelerates in the fourth and fifth decades and gathers yet more speed after age 60, requiring greater defensive efforts against aging as we get older.
8. The natural healing powers within us, if properly used, can improve longevity.
9. Mother Nature will help us if we let her.
10. 100 is a good age to strive for, for starters.

Objectives of the Book

Now that we know we *can* live longer, what is in this book that is going to help you do it? We will present key information on:

1. The latest medical information on living a longer, healthier life, discussed in simple terms.
2. Medical facts considered by consensus of the collective wisdom of large medical organizations and the general medical community as non-controversial and positively helpful in achieving longevity.
3. Discussions of the pros and cons of treatments that are not universally accepted, as well as balanced, objective recommendations.
4. The best ways to eat the right foods at home, in restaurants, and at fast food places, to help you remain healthy and live longer.
5. Exercises you can (and should) do at any age with safety and profitability in your bed, living room or office, at a mall or outdoors.
6. Data on factors that affect health and aging such as smoking and other environmental chemicals.
7. Delineations of what is good and what is not throughout your life so you can build a healthful life and live longer.
8. Discussions emphasizing how common sense, combined with the use of scientific facts, can go a long way in the fight against aging.
9. Guides to help you feel better, look younger, function better physically and mentally, and live longer: to at least 100 years.
10. And finally, *100 prescriptions* to do this.

The Big Question

Why should we believe that we can live to be 100, or more?

1. Many humans have lived longer. In fact, there are about 70,000 centenarians in the U.S. telling us they did it. Join the next group: it is estimated there will be about 200,000 centenarians in the U.S. by the year 2020 and about 9 million Americans will be over 85.
2. The oldest documented person, Jeanne Louise Calment, lived to be 122 years old. *The Guinness Book of World Records* (1998),

Introduction

TABLE 1.1

Life Expectancies Worldwide

In Ancient Greece	17 years
In Ancient Rome	22 years
In 1776	<40 years
In 1900	47 years
In 1920	54 years
In 1940	63 years
In 1960	69.85 years
In 1970	70.5 years
In 1980	73.7 years
In 1990	75.3 years

notes that she was born on February 21, 1875 and died in France on August 4, 1997.
3. Not far behind is living proof: Marie Louise Febronie, who was born on August 29, 1880, is still kicking away in Canada (Guinness Book of World Records, 1998).
4. Simply "eliminating the top ten causes of death (just by itself) would increase the life expectancy of people over the age of 65 by about 20 years," notes the American Geriatrics Society's *Guide to Aging and Health* (Bortz, 1996).
5. It has been calculated that if the health habits of the past few years continue, in the year 2080, the average life expectancy in America will be 100 years for men and 103 years for women (Manton, 1996). With superior health habits, we believe we will do much better, sooner.
6. Here is another promising prediction. "If the average rate of decrease in death rates continues to prevail in the coming years, in 2050 the average life expectancy will be 100" (Bortz, 1996).

TABLE 1.2

Life Expectancy at 65, United States

Year	Years of Life > 65 Male	Years of Life > 65 Female
1900	11.00	12.00
1920	12.00	12.30
1940	11.90	13.40
1960	12.9	15.90
1980	14.00	18.40
1990	15.20	18.80
2000	15.70	20.80
2010	16.10	21.30
2030	16.80	22.20
2050	17.60	23.10

7. The French biologist, George Buffoon, says the body is built to last: "We have the potential to live six times as long as it took our bones to fully form. The adult skeleton is fully developed at age twenty. Multiply twenty by six and you have one hundred twenty, or one million hours" (Hayflick, 1994).
8. Currently we are realizing only about five-sixths (83.3 %) of our maximum life potential. The U.S. Census Bureau tells us that the fastest growing segment of the population is persons over the age of 100. Utilizing our maximum potential, we can join the higher ranks.
9. Even biblical references indicate that we can live to the age of 120 years. Genesis 6:3 (New Jerusalem Bible translation) states, "My spirit cannot be indefinitely responsible for human beings, who are only flesh; let the time allowed be a hundred and twenty years."

Introduction

10. A historical view of life expectancy predicts that people will continue to live longer. This trend is clear in Tables 1.1 and 1.2. There is no doubt these numbers will change for the better.

The Goal of this Book is to Help You Live Longer

Now: **One life = ¾ of a century**
One life = 75 years
One life = 7.5 decades
One life = 300 seasons
One life = 900 months
One life = 3,600 weeks
One life = 25,200 days
One life = 604,800 hours
One life = 36,288,000 minutes
One life = 2,177,280,000 seconds

One life = 3,155,414,400 seconds
One life = 52,590,240 minutes
One life = 876,504 hours
One life = 36,521 days
One life = 5,218 weeks
One life = 1200 months
One life = 400 seasons
One life = 10 decades
One life = 100 years

Goal: **One life = One century**

...or, a longer, healthier life. You can do it. Read on. We have found ways to do it. We have 100 prescriptions for you to live to be 100.

References

Bortz, W.M. (1996). *Dare to Be 100.* New York, NY: Simon and Schuster.

Guinness Book of World Records. (1998). Stanford, CT: Guinness Media, Inc.

Hayflick, L. (1994). *How and Why We Age.* New York, NY: Ballantine Books.

Manton, K.G., et al. (1996). Longevity in the United States: Age and sex-specific evidence on life-span limits from mortality patterns 1960-1990. *Journal of Gerontology: Biological Sciences, 5 I A*, B362.

Chapter 2

Primary Prescriptions: Ten Health Commandments

Commandment I.   Thou shalt eat healthy.

Commandment II.   Thou shalt exercise.

Commandment III.   Thou shalt not smoke or use any harmful substances.

Commandment IV.   Thou shalt watch thy weight and care for thy body.

Commandment V.   Thou shalt stay active mentally and physically.

Commandment VI.   Thou shalt reduce thy level of stress.

Commandment VII.   Thou shalt be informed, believe in thy power to heal thyself.

Commandment VIII.   Thou shalt seek peace.

Commandment IX.   Thou shalt love.

Commandment X.   Thou shalt do something positive for thy health every day

These are primary prescriptions. In order to fully get the best out of these prescriptions, succeeding chapters present the information and practical advice for you. Simple lists of facts cover all important aspects of longevity. The discussion will lead you to 100 prescriptions to help you live to be 100, in good health.

Chapter 3

Ten Storytellers in Their Nineties: Their Gold Standards and Prescriptions for Longevity

In this chapter we present interviews of ten randomly selected patients and friends, all in their nineties, one from each year. The following summaries of the conversations with them unfold some remarkable stories that make it clear why they have lived long. Their stories are power packs of good advice and a large deck of the golden rules of life. To top it all off, they contribute their *prescriptions* for longevity.

J.B. — Age 90

A friend, a neighbor, and sometimes a walking companion, J.B., who has an arched back, goes around our block in a shuffling gait, with his dog on a leash. He says he has always been physically active. Now retired, he does all of the housework, leaving no chores for his daughter with whom he lives. His daily routine consists of cleaning floors, washing dishes, polishing furniture, a lot of yard work and walking. Recently he painted the exterior of his home: he's not afraid to climb ladders.

J.B. is a true "work-liker" (he does not like the word "workaholic"). His working history began at age 8 when he sold newspapers. He says he had to work to support his family. At the age 15 he continued, doing a lot of physical work for a construction company. His sincere hard work took him to a supervisory position. While he did this full-time job, he also ran his candy store, at night and on weekends. Even when he was drafted during World War II for the Defense Department, he did extra part-time jobs working until midnight.

J.B. eats lots of fruits. At home he eats a low-fat diet but in restaurants he goes for everything—milk, ice cream, fried foods. He loves chicken, drinks soda everyday, and half a glass of wine two to three times a week. He does all the grocery shopping himself.

He is extremely articulate and mentally alert. He reads newspapers, magazines and watches only *The Wheel of Fortune*, *Jeopardy* and news on television. He prays at home every night and goes to church on Sundays. He wears hearing aids but his vision is good and his overall health is excellent. He takes no medications and has never used vitamin supplements. His recent medical check up and tests gave him a clean bill of health.

When asked to give a *prescription for longevity*, he leaned forward and said, "Listen carefully. Walk, eat right, and don't smoke. Stay excited; always think about the next day. But, the most important thing is—stay busy."

M.M. — Age 91

Born in a small town in India, M.M. got his medical degree at the age of 23. He specialized in Ophthalmology and taught and practiced eye surgery in India until the mandatory retirement age of 58. He has not stopped being physically and mentally active, now devoting his time to social work, reading, writing and traveling. He spends much of his time in the U.S. with his wife, children and grandchildren.

Talking of his family history he says: "I was very unfortunate to see my father die at the very young age of 76. My mother died at 90. If you live right you don't have to die that early." The "right life," M.M. believes, means you, "Work hard, but keep stress away. As a physician I worked two to three times more than an average person did, but it was all positive stress because I enjoyed every minute of the work time. I was a 'people person'. For the ultimate in life, I came home where the love of my wife and other family members kept me ignited all the time. Be helpful and kind to others and peace will be yours. With my kind of right life, you will be gifted with good, sound sleep every night." In a priestly tone he continued, "Integrity and honesty are important. Live a dream life. Give. Love. Pray."

Just as his parents did, M.M. walks a lot. They were very religious and so is M.M. He prays every day. His parents were strict vegetarians and so is M M. His diet includes a lot of vegetables, fruits, and whole grain preparations with minimal fat.

To date M.M.'s health is excellent. Except for occasional bouts of allergy symptoms, he is doing well. He looks great and dresses well. He is totally in charge of his life. He shows up for medical check ups regularly. His blood pressure is normal, his latest cholesterol reading is 200, HDL 50 and LDL 125. He proudly says, "There is no current threat of ill health or disability."

His *prescription for longevity*: "Peace of mind, and good sleep."

E.A. — Age 92

"What is your wish, E.A.?" We asked her. "I just want to look good." In fact, she looks great every time she visits our office—with matching clothes, perfect make up, and nice jewelry. She walks briskly and speaks swiftly and articulately.

At 5'2", she weighs 125 lbs. She has the blood pressure of a teenager and good blood chemistry. Her health is excellent.

"How do you account for your good health, E.A.?" She replies: "I walk a lot, with no arthritis to limit me. I eat a lot of vegetables and fruits and they make my skin look good. I live an up life and am never depressed."

E.A. had her share of tragedies in her life. One husband died after 43 years of marriage, and another after 11 1/2 years of marriage. "I am still thanking the Lord for those lovely years. You want to be happy? Forget the negatives of life, thrive on the positives. I carry those positives to bed and sleep like a baby for seven hours every night, and nap some days."

Her *prescription*: "There is nothing wrong in life. If you keep thinking that way, then there will be nothing wrong in the future."

R.P — Age 93

A "social butterfly" with several close friends, R.P. loves to talk about the simplicity of her life. She lives alone and enjoys her independence. She says with confidence, "I don't need any help from any one; I drive, so I can go anywhere any time. I do my own grocery shopping, run errands and go any place I want to. When I am at home, I do all the cooking, cleaning and check writing."

This modified lifestyle started when her husband died after 57 years of "fantastic" marriage. "The only thing he did wrong to me was that he smoked," she says, adding, "If he hadn't, he would not have left me so early." During their marriage R.P. was always a homemaker, working hard at it.

The following are the "simple facts" of her lifestyle that she believes have kept her healthy:

Diet: She has a waffle or cereal and tea for breakfast every day at about 7:00 am. She eats a heavy lunch with chicken or fish (no red meat) with vegetables and coffee. A cookie with tea in the mid-afternoon and usually a sandwich for dinner. Another snack, cookie or cereal if she is hungry before going to bed.

Exercise: R.P. swims one hour every morning, weather permitting. She walks one to two miles every day and she goes dancing every weekend: "Some fast dancing, some slow." She has never smoked and has never used alcohol. For recreation, R.P. reads a lot, and watches some television. She plays bingo two to three times a week. Every morning she prays, and goes to church every Sunday. She sleeps about six hours per night.

R.P is in perfect health, except for mild hypertension. She has good hearing and good eyesight. She is 5'1" and weights 104 pounds, and has never weighed more than 115 pounds.

When asked about her *prescription for longevity*, she came up with several: "Work hard. Eat right. Don't eat junk food. Avoid desserts. Be patient with others. Be happy with what you have. Don't worry about tomorrow."

R.P. — Age 94

At introduction, when she shook hands, I felt R.P. was going to crush my bones to pieces. I grinned. She laughed and said, "I'm a southpaw, watch out." All of her relatives are dead. She lives in a nursing home.

After getting a college degree she worked as a teacher. She said, "I never wanted to retire, but they forced me to at 70." She has not slowed down, she bounces around socializing all day. She has a lot of friends and entertains them by playing the piano. She said, "I have a great life, and helping others makes it better."

"How is your lifestyle?" She responded: "Great, I am active. I don't smoke. I take a highball now and then. I was born on a farm, so I love vegetables and fruits. I eat some chicken and fish, but rarely meat. I never took any vitamins. I sleep soundly all night."

She has been perfectly healthy all her life, and has never needed any medications. Aside from two c-sections she has had no surgeries.

When asked about her secret *formula for longevity* she advised: "Live a good clean life, be generous, and help others."

F.H. — Age 95

He is trim and mentally sharp. Every statement he makes is full of humor. F.H. says: "I started working at age nine, small jobs in the beginning, truck driver in between, I was a tavern owner for 30 years, and retired at 70. But, I still have three hobbies: 1. Work, 2. Work, 3. Work."

F.H. has been physically active all his life. He has done a lot of walking during his life. His wife said, "He always walks like a rabbit." Now he does most of his walking in the malls, about two to three miles every day. "I was born with a cigar in my mouth. I am 95 and the cigar is still there in my mouth but now I just chew it. Never touched cigarettes. I eat anything and everything. I love soup. I drink skim milk every day. I have never missed a breakfast in my life and it has always been a good big meal."

F.H. has been healthy all his life. He is a very compliant patient and never misses an appointment for his check up. During a recent visit, he had no complaints, his examination was negative, his EKG was normal and laboratory tests showed cholesterol at 165, triglycerides 120, glucose 95 and PSA 0.3—all normal.

He has been married for 49 years and sexually active until the age of 90. "My marriage has been damn good," he said, and quickly adds his *prescription for longevity*: "The best way to live long is to get a good wife."

M.T. — Age 96

At his age, M.T. has an unusual flare for talking. He is precise with his words and clear in his thinking. During our interview in the retirement home, he kept pacing with his walker while talking. He stopped near a piano and said, "I love music." He regularly plays music. His other hobbies are photography and reading.

M.T. is an orthodox Jew. He went to a Hebrew school. He still has a sharp mind. He organizes and conducts all religious ceremonies on all holidays for the residents of the retirement home. He emphasizes, "Pray and you will live long."

M.T. is lucky to carry good longevity genes. He said, "My mother would have lived to be a hundred if she were not killed in an accident at 86. And my father would not have died from appendicitis at 69 if antibiotics were available. My daughters are very healthy, thank God, at 65 and 62." He had a "very successful and happy" marriage. His wife died in 1986 and he still misses her a lot. He graduated from high school 80 years ago. He worked hard and built a large transportation business.

M.T. has high blood pressure and cancer of the prostate. Both are under control at this time. He fractured his hip in 1997, and then again in 1998. But nothing has slowed him down. He still exercises regularly.

He quit smoking 40 years ago because of "one bout of bronchitis." He does not use alcohol, and his diet consists mainly of fruits, vegetables, chicken and fish. He has never taken vitamins.

When questioned about the *salient elements of his longevity* M.T. responded: "In summary: a good business, a good marriage, good children, and God."

R.C — Age 97

When she showed up for our interview, R.C. was beautifully attired in color-coordinated clothes and meticulous make-up. The retirement home staff told us that she is always dressed well. She walked to us with brisk, confident steps without a walker or cane. Bespectacled, but with good vision and hearing, she did not once ask to repeat the questions posed to her. Amazingly alert, her responses were quick and to the point.

She worked in the insurance industry from age 17 to age 64. In retirement, she worked even longer hours "helping others." She is very active even now and said, "I don't like to miss my exercises. I do them a full hour, three times a week." She used to swim a lot, but has slowed down now.

R.C. says: "I have always been healthy. Ten years ago they removed a tumor from my colon. No big deal! I've had no problems since then. I go for a check-up every year. During the last check-up a few months ago, my doctor didn't find a single thing wrong with me. Blood pressure, sugar, cholesterol, everything normal." R.C. never had a pap smear. She said she didn't need one, because she never married and had no children. She has never had a mammogram either. She is not on any medications and does not use any vitamin supplements. She has never smoked.

"What about your diet?" Responding to this question she said, "I eat everything. Coffee, a banana, orange juice and toast with margarine for breakfast. A sandwich, soup, grapefruit and skim milk for lunch. And for dinner, a salad, chicken (often), beef (occasionally) or fish (rarely), soup and skim milk. I never eat snacks and I never drink soft drinks, but I have a cocktail (scotch) occasionally."

R.C. comments: "I have lived a simple life. I have always been happy. I never complain. I don't hurt people. I help if I can. I sleep for seven hours at night, and take an afternoon nap sometimes."

About her *prescription for longevity* she said, "Work, even if you retire. Help others."

C.H — Age 98

C.H. is one of our most beloved patients. He makes his own appointments, always comes on time, each time immaculately dressed in jacket and tie. A pure and sweet smile always lights up his face. His medical complaints are usually minor. His trim physique is enviable—no kyphosis, no saggy skin, no trace of obesity. He speaks clearly with polished language.

How did C.H. amass all the life's attributes, including confidence, mental alertness, physical integrity, good health and good manners? He has a two-word formula: "balanced life."

Born in Sweden, C.H. came to the U.S. in 1923. He conscientiously climbed the ladder of success to end up as a superintendent of a large construction company. He retired from that job at age 64 because "it was a nerve-racking job with high pressure." However, physically he did not slow down. He played golf every day until he was 95 and since then he has become a shuffleboard addict. He swims a half-hour every day. To stay mentally active C.H. reads magazines, newspapers and watches news on television.

C.H. eats "lots of salads and fruits," with chicken or fish; no red meats, no alcohol. He does not smoke. He has a lot of friends. He sleeps one to two hours in the day time and eight to nine hours at night. He, too, has good longevity genes. His father died at 95, and his mother at 80. He has three siblings in their eighties. His recent EKG was perfectly normal, and so were his blood tests: glucose 93, cholesterol 152 and triglycerides 76.

C.H.'s *prescription for longevity*: "Hard work, clean life, balanced diet."

Y.L. — Age 99

"How did you make it to 99 Y.L.?" Jokingly she raised her right hand with a glass and said "This," (martinis) and raised her left hand with a cigarette and said "This." More seriously she comments: "Both of these things would have destroyed my immune system but I did a thousand other good things that kept it revived!"

Y.L. used to have two martinis before dinner. She used to smoke up to four packs of cigarettes per day, and still has to have two packs daily. As she says: "I am addicted to smoking but I am not addicted to nicotine. I don't inhale smoke, period."

Knowing that I am a pathologist, when she walked into my office unassisted with her 74-year-old son (funeral director), she jabbed again, "Are you two going to put me away or what?"

This amazing lady was a business tycoon. She owned and operated 35 beauty shops in Boston, and ran a weight loss program on a place called "The Fat Farm."

She has her own set ways even now. She sleeps ten to twelve hours every night, getting up only once to go to the bathroom, and she naps for two hours in the afternoon. She eats three good meals a day but does not eat snacks, desserts, and does not drink soft drinks. She has to have two capsules of garlic every day. She enjoys tea in the morning and afternoon. Remarkably, she is still physically active; walks around her oceanfront apartment and swims every day alone in the shallow end of the pool. She prays daily and watches religious shows on television on Sundays. She needs no assistance for any of her domestic activities.

Y.L. is a gambler and travels to Freeport, Bahamas every week. She takes along a fixed gambling budget of $500 and wins more often than not.

About her health, she says: "I have no disease, I am in perfect health and I am happy, and I am going to live long." Her last check up was impressive. Everything was normal, including the EKG, cholesterol 186, triglycerides 74, HDL 83, LDL 88 and glucose 86. She weighs 100 pounds.

Y.L.'s *prescription for longevity*: "Keep a positive attitude. Be in charge. I have been a boss lady all my life, so I know it."

These stories have a lot of "meat" in them. Some of the persons interviewed urged us to distribute this meaningful information to benefit others. The balance of the book is all about disseminating their messages, our messages, and scientific facts that would be helpful to anyone who wants to live a long and healthy life.

Section II.

The Critical Role of Diet

Chapter 4

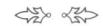

⊰⊱ ⊰⊱

Foods for Longevity: Things You Must Know

Let us start with COMMANDMENT I, *Thou shalt eat healthy.* To obey this commandment, we must first understand what the bounty of Nature is and identify the components of that bounty that are essential for our survival: the foods necessary for survival and longevity.

i. Protein: Pound for Pound the Best Power Booster

"Protein is who you are," says Walter M. Bortz II (1996) and he isn't exaggerating. This organic substance comprises 60% of our non-water weight. It is the main ingredient of our brains, muscles and hearts. In fact, the word comes from the Greek *proteios*, meaning "of prime importance." Here are *ten life-lengthening facts about protein*:

1. Protein is made up of 20 amino acids, which are in turn comprised of carbon, nitrogen, hydrogen, oxygen and a bit of sulfur. Since the human body cannot produce nine of these amino acids, they must be included in the diet.
2. Protein is the body's main building material, responsible for making bones, teeth, skin, nerves, muscles, blood components, anti-bodies and serving as an energy source for the metabolic activity of each cell.

TABLE 4.1

Daily Protein Requirement

Ideal Weight	Protein Needed	Safety Margin
80 lb	40 g	50 g
111 lb	50 g	60 g
120 lb	55 g	65 g
133 lb	60 g	70 g
156 lb	70 g	80 g
167 lb	75 g	85 g
178 lb	80 g	90 g
200 lb	90 g	100 g
222 lb	100 g	110 g
244 lb	110 g	120 g

3. At four calories per gram, protein is a weight-conscious source of energy and heat when carbohydrates and fats are unavailable. If protein is used in place of these nutrients, however, it can't perform its primary function of building and protecting tissues. This can compromise health. All items must be used together.
4. Protein molecules, or enzymes, are the catalyst for hundreds of chemical reactions, including energy storage and nutrient synthesis.
5. Protein requirements vary with body weight. For instance, a 120 lb person needs about 55 g per day and a 200 lb person needs about 90 g per day. For more details, see Table 4.1.
6. The expression "too much of a good thing" applies to protein. Most Americans eat far more than they need, and the excess is stored as fat. What's more, excess protein creates extra work for the liver and kidneys. It is broken down and processed by these organs.

7. Healthy high-protein foods include eggs, fish, lean meat, legumes and low fat milk.
8. Seniors need to pay extra attention to their protein consumption to help guard against muscle loss.
9. The protein values of some common foods are: three ounces of sirloin steak–26 g; three ounces of flounder–20 g; eight ounces of whole milk–8 g; one ounce of American cheese–6 g; one large egg–6 g.

ii. Carbohydrates: The Fast Lane Energizer

"Whether you are an athlete, a diabetic, or a heart patient, if you are suffering from high blood pressure or obesity, or are just a healthy person interested in staying that way, a diet that is high in fiber and complex carbohydrates is your best bet for living long and well," says health writer Jane Brody (1985). These ten fast facts about carbohydrates will show you why:

1. As a dietary source of sugar, carbohydrates are the body's main source of energy. They also promote the storage of muscle fuel and help digestion.
2. Foods high in complex carbohydrates contain a variety of vitamins and minerals and are low in calories.
3. Carbohydrates are an essential component of any diet and they should form the bulk of your diet.
4. Carbohydrate deficiencies deprive the brain of serotonin, an important chemical that affects mood and sleep.
5. Carbohydrates are an excellent food for dieting. They cause extra calories to be burned. They contain less than half the calories of fat. And their fiber is so filling that you tend to eat less.
6. Carbohydrates help reduce the risk of cancer, particularly of the colon.
7. Try to avoid refined carbohydrates, the highly processed and low-fiber variety in white flour, candies, carbonated beverages and white sugar. These enter the bloodstream and are absorbed more quickly than complex carbohydrates, making for a quick energy "fix". This is followed by a hunger for more. Choose complex carbohydrates:

vegetables, fruits, and whole grains are the best sources. Refer to Tables 4.4 and 4.5.
8. If you notice an increase in flatulence and bloating as you add complex carbohydrates to your diet, control it by increasing your intake gradually.
9. The American Heart Association recommends a carbohydrate intake of 55–60% or more of total calories.
10. To get the amount of carbohydrate you need, eat 6–11 servings a day of grain foods (meat, cereals, pasta, rice), 2–4 servings of fruit and 3–5 servings of vegetables.

iii. Fat: Store It, Use It, But Don't Overdo It

Fat is an essential component of a diet. One gram of fat gives nine calories. A healthy person should get fewer than 30% of total calories from fat. Your calorie level will determine how much fat you should include in your diet.

But be careful about the type of fat you eat. There are two main types of fat: saturated fatty acids and unsaturated fatty acids. The latter are divided into polyunsaturated and monounsaturated. Simply put, saturated fats raise the levels of total cholesterol and bad cholesterol (LDL) and therefore are bad for the heart. Reducing the intake of saturated fats and cholesterol is the best way to lower your total cholesterol and bad cholesterol (LDL) and reduce the risk of coronary artery disease.

So, how much of each type of fat is appropriate for a healthy person who wants to reduce the risk of coronary heart disease? Prudently follow the American Heart Association (AHA) guidelines. Limit the saturated fatty acid intake to 8–10% of total calories. To reduce the amount of saturated fatty acids, avoid coconut oil and butter, trim all the fat from the meats you eat and remove all the skin from poultry. A glance at Table 4.2 will tell you the percentages of saturated, monounsaturated, and polyunsaturated fats in different oils.

If you want to lower high blood cholesterol, follow the Step I and Step II diets devised by the AHA and The National Cholesterol Education Program discussed in Chapter Five.

TABLE 4.2
Ten Good & Bad Oils

Oil/Fat	Saturated	Monounsaturated	Polyunsaturated
Canola Oil	7%	60%	30%
Safflower Oil	9%	13%	76%
Corn Oil	13%	25%	59%
Olive Oil	14%	76%	9%
Soybean Oil	15%	24%	59%
Peanut Oil	17%	47%	32%
Margarine	20%	48%	32%
Plus three to avoid:			
Coconut Oil	89%	6%	2%
Butter	64%	29%	4%
Veg. Shortening	25%	45%	20%

iv. Cholesterol: Careful Concern

A healthy body needs cholesterol. It serves several functions:

1. It contributes to the synthesis of hormones.
2. It protects the integrity of cell membranes.
3. It contributes to the formation of bile salts.
4. It improves the health of skin and nails.
5. It helps the nerves to send messages.

Then, why is cholesterol bad? Too much cholesterol in the blood contributes to arteriosclerosis, the hardening of the arteries, which leads to heart attacks. Your liver produces most of the cholesterol, about 1,000 mg per day. But you get some from your food. Most of it comes from meats, eggs, poultry, fish and dairy products. Table 4.3 shows different food items and the amounts of cholesterol in each. There is low cholesterol in fruits, vegetables, and grains.

Blood cholesterol level is a measure to determine your risk of heart disease. A level of 200 mg/dl or less is considered to be "normal" or "good", associated with low risk. The level between 200 and 240 mg/dl is considered a moderate risk and the level higher than 240 mg/dl is considered a high risk for heart disease.

The chemicals that transport cholesterol across blood vessels are called lipoproteins. There are four types of lipoproteins:

1. Chlyomicrons
2. Very low density lipoproteins (VLDL)
3. Low density lipoproteins (LDL)
4. High density lipoproteins (HDL)

The HDL carries cholesterol out of the blood vessels and is commonly described as "good cholesterol" and the VLDL and LDL transport cholesterol into the blood vessels and are called "bad cholesterol". So, the higher the level of the HDL the better it is and the lower the level of LDL the better it is. A level of less than 130 mg/dl of the LDL is considered normal. High levels of the LDL increase the risk of heart attacks. Exercise and alcohol consumption in moderation increases the level of HDL. A diet high in saturated fats increases the level of cholesterol and LDL thus increasing the chances of hardening of the arteries.

v. Fruits: Oh, so Heavenly

We can't think of a good reason why a person would not meet the daily recommendations for fruit intake. They taste good, are easily available and provide an enormous health benefit. The good news is there are hundreds of types of fruits and fruit juices. The United States Department of Agriculture developed the Food Pyramid as a guide for people to optimize

TABLE 4.3
Cholesterol in Commonly Used Foods

Food	Serving Size	Cholesterol
Large egg	1	213 mg
Butter	1 pat	11 mg
Whole milk	1 cup	33 mg
2 % milk	1 cup	18 mg
1 % milk	1 cup	18 mg
Skim milk	1 cup	10 mg
Cheese (American)	1 oz	27 mg
Cheese (Cheddar)	1 oz	30 mg
Cheese (Cream)	1 oz	31 mg
Cheese (Mozzarella, whole milk)	1 oz	22 mg
Cheese (Mozzarella, skim milk)	1 oz	15 mg
Cheese (Swiss)	1 oz	26 mg
Potato, baked	N/A	0 mg
Rice	N/A	0 mg
Groud Beef, reg. / Sirloin Steak	3 oz	77 mg
Chicken Breast	3 oz	73 mg
Salmon (baked)	3 oz	60 mg
Pasta	N/A	0 mg

TABLE 4.4
Ten Best Fruits

Item	Serving Size	KCal	Fat g	Protein g	Carb g	Fiber g	Vit A re	Vit C mg
Apple	1	125	0.8	0.4	32	6.58	11	12
Apricots	3	51	0.4	1.5	11.8	2.23	277	10.6
Banana	1	105	0.5	1.2	26.7	3.26	9	10
Blueberries	1 c	82	0.6	1	20.5	4.93	15	20
Blackberries	1 c	82	0.6	1	20.5	4.93	15	20
Grapefruit	½	37	0.1	0.7	9.4	1.53	32	47
Grapes	10	35	0.3	0.3	8.9	1	4	5
Orange	1	60	0.2	1.2	15.4	2.97	27	70
Pear	1	98	0.7	0.7	25.1	4.98	3	7
Strawberries	1 c	45	0.6	0.9	10.5	3.28	4	85

their nutritional intake (see Chapter 5). In that, the amount of fruit suggested is 2–4 servings per day. That is equivalent to one medium sized fruit such as an apple, banana or orange; 1/4 cup of dried fruit such as prunes, apricots or raisins; six ounces of fruit juice.

Fruits have it all. They are low in fat, low in cholesterol, low in calories, high in fiber, high in vitamins, minerals and water. All of these aspects are beneficial to your health. In addition, they are good sources of antioxidants. It is known that foods high in fiber can contribute to longevity. That is because fiber decreases heart disease by lowering cholesterol. It also acts to decrease colon cancer by improving absorption in the intestines. Antioxidants have been considered cancer fighters because they prevent the action of free radicals which damage cells. Vitamins of course are necessary for the everyday functioning of our bodies, and folate is necessary especially for pregnant women, to decrease the chance of an infant developing a neurological birth defect. Fruits provide all of these essential nutrients.

So start the day not with coffee but with a glass of juice. At lunch time, opt for a fruit juice instead of a carbonated drink. A fruit can make an ideal snack or dessert. Make a change for the better, eat fruit. Table 4.4 lists the ten best.

vi. Vegetables: Mother Nature's Greatest Gifts

Vegetables are beneficial to a person's health, and contribute to longevity. They are low in fat, cholesterol and calories, high in vitamins and minerals, high in antioxidants and rich in fiber. For the ten best see Table 4.5.

The Food Guide Pyramid (see Chapter 6) recommends eating three to five servings of vegetables a day. Examples of one serving are:

1 cup salad	½ cup canned vegetables
1 ear of corn on the cob	1 medium tomato
3 to 5 spears of broccoli	8 baby carrots
6 spears of asparagus	

If you are a vegetarian, you can meet your daily nutritional requirements. Just follow the food guide pyramid. To create a balanced vegetarian meal, combine three to five servings of vegetables (cooked or raw vegetables 1/2 cup and raw leafy vegetables 1 cup) with two to four servings of fruit, two to three servings of beans, nuts, seeds and one to three servings of milk, yogurt, cheese (American Dietetic Association, 1997).

Vegetables are natural products and they require a good washing before eating. There is not a significant difference in nutritional value between fresh, frozen or canned vegetables. They contain only traces of fat, mainly unsaturated fatty acids. Vegetables contain two of the best antioxidants, vitamin C and vitamin E. Vegetables rich in antioxidants are: carrots, broccoli, sweet potatoes. Cruciferous vegetables contain large amounts of vitamin C, fiber and antioxidants.

TABLE 4.5
Ten Best Vegetables

Item	Serving Size	KCal	Fat g	Protein g	Carb g	Fiber g	Vit A re	Vit C mg
Broccoli	1	24	0.3	2.6	4.6	3	136	8
Cabbage	1 c	16	0.1	0.8	3.8	1.6	9	33
Carrots	1 c	30	0.1	0.7	7	2	202	7
Cauliflower	½ c	12	0.0	1	2.5	1.3	0	36
Corn Cob	1	83	1	2.6	19	3.6	17	5
Onion	1 c	54	0.4	1.9	11.7	2.6	0	13
Green Pepper	½	12	0.2	0.4	2.6	1.07	261	76
Potato	1	220	0.2	4.7	51	4.4	0	26
Soybeans	1 c	235	10.2	19.8	19.5	4	5	0
Tomato	1 c	35	0.4	1.6	7.8	3	204	32

vii. Grains: Bread, Cereals and Flours for You

"Give us this day our daily bread." In Western culture, bread is a symbol for nourishment. In the Orient, it is rice. *Ten grainy facts about grain products* will show how they earned their superb reputation:

1. According to the Food Guide Pyramid, a healthy adult's diet should consist of 6–11 servings of bread, pasta and other grain products. One serving equals one slice of bread or about one cup of pasta or rice.
2. Grains are low-priced, easy to cook and extremely nutritious. They are rich in protein, low in fat, and abundant in vitamins and minerals, fiber and complex carbohydrates.

TABLE 4.6
Ten Best Grains

Item	Serving Size	KCal	Fat g	Protein g	Carb g	Fiber g	Vit A re	Vit C mg
All Bran®	1/3	70	0.5	4	21	8.4	375	15
GrapeNuts®	1/2	202	0.2	6.6	26.4	3.31	753	0
Cornflakes	1	211	1.8	5.3	52.7	5.8	500	0
Shredded Wheat	3/4 c	115	0.8	3.5	25	3.9	0	0
Wheaties®	1	101	0.5	2.8	23.1	3.3	388	15
Brown Rice	1	232	1.2	5	50	4	0	0
Whole Wheat	1	400	2.4	16	85	15.2	0	0
Cheerios®	1	89	1.4	3.4	15.7	0.9	304	12
Barley	1	190	0.0	4.0	44	4.4	0	0
Oatmeal	1	145	2.0	6	25	9.2	4	0

3. For good health, plan your meals around grains. Serve meats and vegetables as side dishes. For the ten best sources of grains, refer to Table 4.6.
4. Whole grains are the most nutritious; refined or white grains are less so. Limit your intake of refined white flours and rices that, after processing, no longer contain most of the vitamins, minerals or fiber they were born with.
5. Rice is a very common food source for over half the world. Westerners tend to equate protein with meat. But in the East, rices are often the primary, and sometimes only, source of protein.
6. Fish is usually considered the best source of heart and health protective omega-3 fatty acids. In fact, whole grains contain omega-3s

that are more likely to produce age-reducing free radicals than is fish oil.
7. To find a healthy loaf of bread, look for "whole" flour bread.
8. For a super high-protein, high-fiber treat, especially for those allergic to wheat, try quinoa (pronounced keen-WA). This was a food staple of the ancient Inca civilization and is making a come back in health-conscious circles. Quinoa supplies a good balance of all essential amino acids and is a far better source of calcium, iron and phosphorus than wheat, yellow corn or white rice.
9. Ordinary pasta is made from processed white flour. Stick to whole wheat-based pastas, including those made with corn, spelt and quinoa.
10. In addition to quinoa, experiment with these other super-charged grains: amaranth, buckwheat groats, bulgar, pearled barley, wild rice, millet, triticale, wheat berries, and good old brown rice.

viii. Beans: Power Pack of Essential Amino Acids

As nations become more prosperous and their citizens have more food, they tend to eat less of the healthy stuff. Take the humble bean, long a staple of both American and Japanese diets, now giving way to steak and hamburger. The more you know about beans, the more likely you are to make them a bigger part of your diet. To that end, check out these reasons to load up on beans:

1. Beans belong to the legume family, which includes lentils, peas and chickpeas. They are high in protein, low in fat, contain no cholesterol, and are a good source of heart-healthy stable Omega-3 fatty acids.
2. Soybeans, known as the "queen of beans," produce more protein per acre than any other thing. The virtues of protein in soybeans are described later in this chapter.
3. Beans are among the few foods besides whole grains that provide thiamine, which helps convert carbohydrates and fats to energy.
4. Another B vitamin, folacin, is found in dried beans. It helps produce nucleic acids responsible for helping with cell division and is important in the production of hemoglobin.

5. Dried beans contain water soluble fibers.
6. Beans are an important source of vitamin E, an antioxidant that helps guard against aging.
7. Iron is another important component of beans.
8. Here's an anti-gas tip from Alfred Olson of the U.S. Department of Agriculture. First, rinse the beans and remove any foreign particles. Then pour boiling water over them and let them soak for at least four hours. Next, toss out the water and cook them in fresh water (Tufts University Health and Nutrition Letter, 1999).
9. A half cup of baked beans has just 160 calories, two to three grams of fat and nine grams of fiber.
10. Nine grams of beans contain almost half the 20 g daily amount of fiber recommended by the National Cancer Institute, and are a power pack of essential amino acids.

ix. Salt: The Vices and Virtues

Salt is vital to life. It is crucial for regulating the body's fluid electrolyte balance and it controls the flow of water and chemicals in and out of the cells. Let us look at *ten important facts about salt*:

1. We need salt but it should be consumed in moderate amounts. The daily intake of sodium should be 2,400 mg. This amount is available in six grams of sodium chloride or salt (approximately 1 1/2 teaspoons).
2. Most Americans consume more salt than they need. This is because they add extra salt to what is already used during food processing and preparation.
3. Salt is everywhere. Canned foods, ketchup, and sauces are heavy in salt. Many people forget that there is salt in alcohol and soft drinks. Read the labels. Look for low-sodium items. Sodium is also present naturally in foods such as natural cheeses, seafish and shellfish.
4. The foods eaten away from home often contain excessive amounts of salt. In the chapters on fast foods and international restaurants you will find the amount of salt in different items.

5. To cut down on salt, consume plenty of fruits and vegetables. They are naturally low in fat and sodium.
6. Sodium plays an important role in the regulation of blood pressure: High sodium intake is associated with high blood pressure.
7. If you have a family history of hypertension or are otherwise at risk for high blood pressure, you can reduce your chances of developing this condition by consuming less salt.
8. If you have high blood pressure, consult your physician and seek specific advice on the amount of salt you should take. For an example of a Low-Salt Diet menu, refer to Chapter 9.
9. High salt intakes may also increase the amount of calcium excreted in urine and thus increase the body's need for calcium.
10. Even for a healthy normal adult, consuming less salt is not harmful, and can be beneficial, if less than 2,400 mg per day.

x. A Few Facts About Water

1. Water, water, everywhere ... even in your body. Your body is made mostly of water: 50-60 percent of it. You could actually survive up to six weeks without food, using your fat stores. However, without water, dehydration would lead to your death in a matter of one week. Each cell in every organ, needs water to work. Water is nutrition, you cannot live without it.
2. Functions of water: Transports nutrients and carries oxygen to body cells. It aids in digestion of food, dissolving nutrients so they can better be absorbed by the body. It also carries waste products out of your body. Water allows for regulation of body temperature; cools the body with perspiration and acts as insulation in the cold. It lubricates joints and moistens eyes, mouth and nose and hydrates the skin. Another important function of water is regulation of filtration of electrolytes across cell walls.
3. Everyone needs a supply of water to replace fluids lost throughout the day: 28–40 oz lost in breath and perspiration, 20–53 oz lost in

urination, 1.5–6 oz lost in feces. It is recommended that a person drink at least 8 eight ounce glasses of water, or about 64 oz total.
4. Need for water increases under the following circumstances:
   a. Vomiting, diarrhea and fever—all of these instances cause excess loss of water.
   b. Pregnancy and breast feeding.
   c. Exercising—your body perspires and thus you lose more water.
   d. Heat exposure
   e. High protein diet—you need more water to help eliminate the extra nitrogen that comes from the protein.
   f. Medications such as diuretics.
5. Water deficiency causes dehydration. Dehydration causes dry mouth, shortness of breath on exertion, muscle spasms and delirium, kidney failure, weakness and inability to stand.
6. Fruits and vegetables provide a high concentration of water, they are made of up to 80–90% water. Decaffeinated drinks like tea and coffee made with water are good sources. Other sources high in water content are cheese, milk, bagel, and even margarine.
7. Dehydration is one of the most frequent causes of hospitalization among people over the age of 65 and 50% of those admitted for dehydration die within one year (American Dietetic Association Website, http://www.eatright.org, 1998).

Our Prescription: Drink plenty of water every day.

xi. Soy: Discover The Joy of Soy

The soy bean is the most eaten plant food in the world. One quarter of the world's population gets its supply of protein from soy. Soy beans provide 30–35% of calories from protein and the composition of soy protein closely resembles animal protein. Soy foods are low in saturated fat and free of cholesterol. Fat in soy is mostly polyunsaturated fat which does not raise cholesterol level. One half cup of soy beans gives 15 g of protein. In addition, soy contains nine amino acids, which are the building blocks of proteins. Soy is high in fiber. This ancient Asian protein source while so popular everywhere has been an unknown in the U.S. for centuries. Only recently it became a nutrition headliner in the U.S. and it is gaining popularity as a food item. The U.S. produces more soybeans than any other country in the world, but most of it is used to feed animals. With its merits as good food, it is bound to be consumed more and more by Americans. The range of soy products in the grocery stores from soy milk to soy cold cuts is an indicator of the change.

1. Soy is heart-healthy. Being low in saturated fat and free of cholesterol it is superior to animal protein. Soy proteins are shown to be lower in total cholesterol by 10–15%. They also lower bad cholesterol (LDL). The good cholesterol level (HDL) remains unchanged. In people with high cholesterol daily consumption of 20–25 g of soy bean protein is shown to lower cholesterol. This amount can be obtained from one cup of soy beans. Soy bean is not only effective in lowering cholesterol level, but it has added merits. It is safe, effective with no side effects observed with the use of cholesterol lowering drugs.
2. Soy may prevent cancer. Soy beans contain several potential anti-cancer substances. The countries which regularly consume soy foods have lower death rates from breast and prostate cancer than the United States. Evidence shows that soy beans are rich in phytochemicals which may lower the risk of several cancers. One serving of soy a day may decrease the risk of several cancers by up to 40%. Half a cup of cooked soy beans or tofu or one cup of soy milk equals a serving.
3. Soy may reduce the risk of osteoporosis. The compounds isoflavones found in soy beans strengthen bones and reduce the risk of osteoporosis.
4. Soy is the best food for diabetics. With moderate amounts of protein, high complex carbohydrates, and low fat, soy becomes

an ideal food for diabetics. It slows absorption of glucose and helps prevent complications of diabetes.
5. Soy beans are available in various forms. Tofu, or bean curd is popularly called the cheese of Asia. Tempeh, popular in Indonesia, is made from cooked whole soy beans. These are nutritious, high fiber foods. Soy milk is a creamy liquid made by boiling soybeans and squeezing out the milk. Soy flour is ground from roasted soy beans. Soy oil is a natural oil extracted from whole soy beans. It is low in saturated fat. Soy sauce is made of soy beans and wheat.

References

American Dietetic Association (1998). Website: http://www.eatright.org.

Bortz, W.M. (1996). *Dare to Be 100.* New York, NY: Simon & Schuster, 104-106.

Brody, Jane E. (1985). *Jane Brody's Good Food Book: Living the High Carbohydrate Way.* New York, NY: W.W. Norton, 18–25.

Dietary fat intake and the risk of coronary heart disease in women. (1997). *New England Journal of Medicine, 337,* 1491–1499.

Hypercholesterolemic and combined hyperlipidemic men. (1997). *Journal of the American Medical Association, 278,* 1509–1515.

Long-term cholesterol lowering effects of 4 fat restricted diets. (1999, April 1). *Tufts University Health and Nutrition Letter, vol. 17, no.2.*

Chapter 5

Ten Famous Diets: Objective Analysis and Advice

The Claims, Contents and Calories
What is Good, What is Not

There are dozens of diets on the market, some good and some bad. Every year more diets are brought into the marketplace and with the power of advertising many do well. Some hold magical control on the population and, despite false or misleading claims, people use them. Most of the diets are targeted at the overweight segment of the population, but some address the issues of good nutrition, lowering of cholesterol levels, and reversal of heart disease.

A good diet has to be medically beneficial to be accepted as good. The value assessment has to be based on the benefits the diet brings. A good diet should produce one or more of the following ten results:

1. It must not be harmful.
2. It should promote health, short term as well as long term.
3. It should provide a medically acceptable number of calories.
4. It should contain medically acceptable amounts of fat, saturated fat, protein and carbohydrate.
5. It should contain adequate amounts of fiber, vitamins and minerals.
6. If it is meant for a certain defined purpose, it should produce the results that improve overall health.
7. Diets targeted for certain diseases should improve conditions, without disturbing the general well being of the persons using them.

8. The diet should have scientifically proven and medically acceptable data justifying the claims.
9. It should be acceptable to the scientific and medical community as safe, effective and beneficial.
10. The diet should combine the merits of good eating and other lifestyle factors generally accepted as health promoting.

We have reviewed numerous "famous" diets. Many that we feel do not meet the above criteria of a good diet have been excluded from discussion. *Ten famous diets* or diet principles considered are presented here. Let us start with a beautiful piece of advice: The Food Pyramid.

i. The Food Pyramid

Principle: The Pyramid, a creation of The United States Department of Agriculture (USDA), incorporates a dietary guideline. It outlines the daily foods with emphasis on eating a variety of foods to get the needed nutrients.

Composition: This is reflected in Diagram 1 (USDA, 1997).

Claims: The food pyramid is not a rigid prescription. It allows a wide selection of items for a healthful diet. It provides all the nutrients you need. It aids in preventing several major diseases.

Servings: It is important to understand what a serving is. A serving in each of the categories reflected in the pyramid is identified below:

Bread, cereal, rice, pasta:
    1/2 cup cooked cereal, rice or pasta, 1 oz cereal, 1 slice bread
Fruits:
    1 medium apple, banana, or orange, 1/2 cup canned fruit, 3/4 cup fruit juice
Vegetables:
    1 cup raw leafy vegetables, 1/2 cup cooked or other raw vegetables, 3/4 cup vegetable juice
Meat, poultry, fish, beans, eggs, nuts:
    2–3 oz lean meat, fish or poultry, 1/2 cup cooked dry beans, 1 egg, 2 Tbl peanut butter

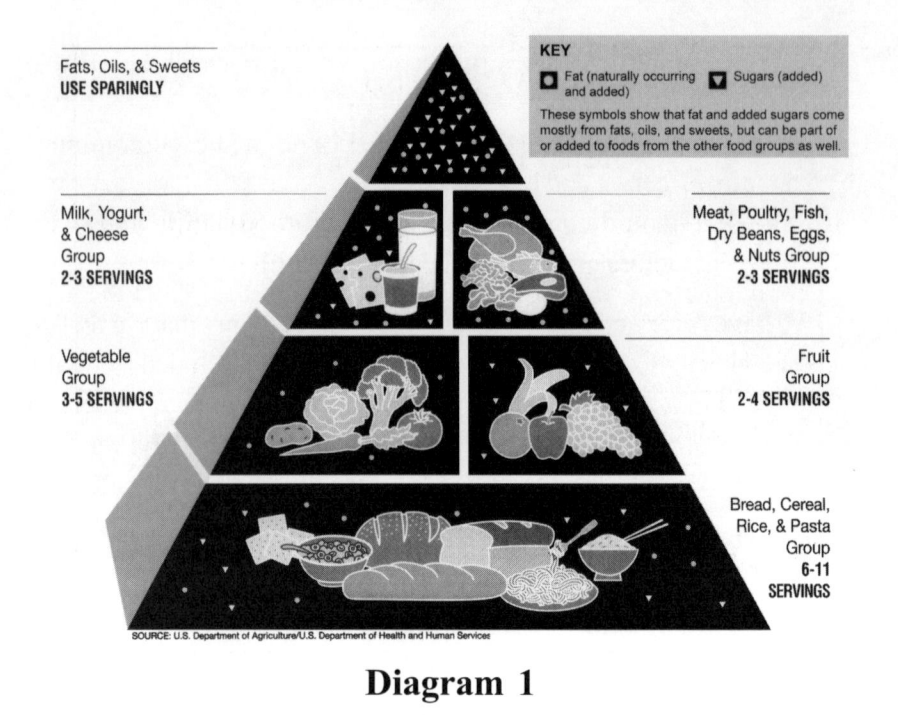

Diagram 1

Food Guide Pyramid:
- Fats, Oils, & Sweets — **USE SPARINGLY**
- Milk, Yogurt, & Cheese Group — **2-3 SERVINGS**
- Meat, Poultry, Fish, Dry Beans, Eggs, & Nuts Group — **2-3 SERVINGS**
- Vegetable Group — **3-5 SERVINGS**
- Fruit Group — **2-4 SERVINGS**
- Bread, Cereal, Rice, & Pasta Group — **6-11 SERVINGS**

KEY: Fat (naturally occurring and added); Sugars (added). These symbols show that fat and added sugars come mostly from fats, oils, and sweets, but can be part of or added to foods from the other food groups as well.

SOURCE: U.S. Department of Agriculture/U.S. Department of Health and Human Services

---

Milk, yogurt, cheese:
   1 cup milk, 1 cup yogurt, 1 1/2 oz natural cheese, 2 oz processed cheese

Advice: The dietary guidelines form a gold-standard, consisting of:

1. A variety of foods
2. Exercise
3. Maintenance of ideal weight
4. Plenty of grains, vegetables and fruits
5. Less fat, saturated fat and cholesterol
6. Moderate amounts of sugar
7. Moderate amounts of sodium and salt
8. Moderate use of alcohol

Calories: Determine appropriate calorie count for your daily diet based on your age and weight.

Update: Major organizations are in the process of revising the federal dietary guidelines for the year 2000 and will advocate a greater role for

TABLE 5.1
Step I Diet Daily Intake

Nutrient	Percentage of Total Calories
Total Fat	< 30%
Saturated Fatty Acids	< 7%
Polyunsaturated Fatty Acids	< 10%
Monounsaturated Fatty Acids	< 15%
Carbohydrate	> 55%
Protein	approx. 15%
Cholesterol	< 200 mg

fruits and vegetables. High intake of fruits and vegetables helps in the prevention of major cancers, coronary artery disease and stroke. It also plays a role in preventing hypertension, asthma, diabetes, obesity, diverticulosis, cataracts and birth defects.

Our comments and prescription: Increase the consumption of fruits and vegetables to reduce the risk of chronic diseases. Add fruit and vegetable juices to daily meals and use more fruits and vegetables as snacks.

ii. Step I. and Step II. Diets

Principle: Step I and Step II diets are for the treatment of high blood cholesterol. The aim of the diets is to reduce the risk of coronary heart disease. The steps have to be carried out under medical supervision.

Composition: (AHA, 1998): For those who have a cholesterol level in excess of 200mg/dl, initial therapy is the Step I diet. This diet consists of 30% or less of total calories from fat. Of these, 8–10% should be derived

TABLE 5.2

Maximum Saturated Fat Intake

Diet Calorie Level	Saturated Fatty Acids
1200 calories	< 9 g
1500 calories	< 12 g
1800 calories	< 14 g
2000 calories	< 16 g
2200 calories	< 17 g
2500 calories	< 19 g
3000 calories	< 23 g

from saturated fatty acids, up to 10% from polyunsaturated fatty acids, and up to 15% from monounsaturated fatty acids. Carbohydrates should provide 55% or more of total calories and proteins, approximately 15%. The daily cholesterol intake should be less than 300 mg/dl. For different calorie levels, the recommended amounts of total fat and saturated fatty acids for the diets are presented in Tables 5.1 and 5.2. The composition of a Step I diet should be as in Table 5.1. For different calorie levels, the recommended Step II diet saturated fatty acid amounts are as in Table 5.2.

Results: Step I diet helps lower the cholesterol level and Step II diet helps achieve further lowering of cholesterol.

Servings: Since Step I and Step II are to be used under medical supervision, your doctor will help you determine the total calorie intake for you to achieve and maintain desired weight. The serving sizes will depend on the number of total calories you need.

Advice: If you have had a heart attack or your cholesterol level is 240mg/dl or higher, start your treatment with the Step II diet. *Follow your doctor's instructions.* Don't forget regular exercises. Lose weight if you are overweight.

Ten Famous Diets: Objective Analysis and Advice   47

Update: Several books contain discussions of Step I and II diets and recipes. The Step I and Step II diets were devised by the American Heart Association (AHA) and the National Cholesterol Education Program (NCEP).

Our comment: These diets are a gold standard of advice. They are produced after considerable discussion and are based on consensus by reputable organizations. This is the best diet advice available for reducing cholesterol levels.

iii. American Cancer Society Diet

Principle: Researchers estimate that about 35% of cancers may be related to diet and suggest that by making simple changes in our eating habits, we can improve our health, help our heart, and reduce the risk of cancer. This is the basis for the American Cancer Society dietary guidelines (Lindsey, 1988).

Composition: The guidelines of the American Cancer Society diet are simple. Less fat, more fiber, lots of vegetable and fruits, moderate intake of alcohol, exercise and maintenance of healthy weight. To cut fats, trim off fat from meats, use less butter, margarine and oil, eat fewer fat–rich desserts and steam, poach, boil or bake foods instead of frying. For fiber go for whole grain cereals, fruits and vegetables. Add fiber with bran, oatmeal, lentils and legumes.

Results: High fat diets have been associated with increased risk of cancers of the colon, rectum, prostate and endometrium. There is also an association, though weaker, between high fat diets and breast cancer. A great deal of evidence indicates that saturated fat may be particularly important in increasing the risk of cancer. Several studies show that the foods rich in antioxidants may lower the risk of cancers of the larynx, esophagus, lung, and bladder. A high fiber diet is also considered possibly protective against cancer.

Servings: The American Cancer Society diet recommendation is for eating five or more servings of fruits or vegetables and six to eleven servings a day of grains and foods made from them. The servings are listed in the preceding section on the Food Pyramid.

Advice: Limit the intake of high fat foods from animal sources and choose most foods from plant sources. With these diet considerations, do regular exercises, maintain a healthy weight and drink alcohol in moderation.

Calories: The daily calorie count can be variable depending on your age and weight. The calorie count is not as important as the composition of the meals.

Update: Recent literature continues to mount indicating that vegetables and fruits reduce the risk of cancer. (For ten best vegetables and legumes refer to Table 4.5, ten best fruits Table 4.4, ten best grains Table 4.6, ten best sources of vitamin A Table 9.1, ten best sources of vitamin E Table 9.3, ten best sources of vitamin C Table 9.2, and for ten best sources of fiber Table 8.2.)

Our advice: This diet is not just good for the prevention of cancer, it is also excellent to reduce the risk of heart disease. The meals allow wide flexibility in the choice of items and all meals can be tasty and enjoyable.

iv. Dr. Dean Ornish's Program for Reversing Heart Disease

Principle: This program has shown that coronary artery disease can be reversed and it can be used as an adjunct to conventional medical therapy. The goal of the program is to help you live longer and feel better even with a serious heart condition.

Composition: The overall program is not just the consideration of diet. It also argues for increased intimacy, reduced stress, regular exercise and no smoking (Ornish, 1990).

Claims/Results:

   a) Within weeks of changing diet, exercising, stress management and group support meetings, the patients reported 91% average reduction in frequency of chest pain. Most became essentially pain free.
   b) On a low fat diet the patients became more insulin sensitive and some were able to stop insulin injections.
   c) There was regression of coronary atherosclerosis. More regression occurred after four to five years in the program than after the first year. In the control group, coronary atherosclerosis continued to progress (Ornish,1999).

Servings: The diet component of the program puts no restrictions on calories. However, the diet must have very low fat, almost no cholesterol, high fiber, and no foods high in saturated fats. The diet allows moderate amounts of salt and sugar, less than two ounces of alcohol per day and inclusion of egg whites in the generally vegetarian diet.

Advice: The program requires total commitment and intensive lifestyle changes such as a low fat vegetarian diet, aerobic exercise, stress management training, smoking cessation and group psychological support.

Menus: The menus reflecting typically vegetarian composition can be found in the book by Dean Ornish.

Calories: This program does not require calorie restriction. Therefore, no calorie counts are needed. This means you can eat as much of the recommended foods as you want.

Results: The latest results reported in *The Journal of the American Medical Association* (1998) indicate that, after five years in the program, patients showed more regression of coronary atherosclerosis than after one year and the number of cardiac events dropped. The control group showed 27.7% worsening of coronary artery blockages after five years.

The American Dietetic Association (ADA) states: "Scientific data suggest positive relationships between a vegetarian diet and reduced risk for several chronic degenerative diseases and conditions, including obesity, coronary artery disease, hypertension, diabetes mellitus, and some types of cancer." (American Dietetic Association Website, 1997).

Our comment: A difficult program to go through, but it certainly produces convincing results.

v. The Pritikin Program for Diet and Exercise:

Principle: The Pritikin Diet is low in fats, cholesterol, protein, and highly refined carbohydrates.

Composition: The average American diet consists of 40–45% calories from fat, 15–20% from protein, and 40–45% from carbohydrates, mostly refined. The Pritikin Diet consists of 5–10% calories from fat, 10–15% from protein and 80% from carbohydrates, mostly complex and unrefined (Pritikin with McGrady, 1979).

Servings: Meat and fish intake restricted to under 1/4 lb daily. Highly refined sugars are banned. Foods high in complex and unrefined carbohydrates, e.g. grains, vegetables, fruits are encouraged. Carry raw vegetables and eat all day long.

Calories: For 600 calories: Three ounces of cooked oatmeal, 3 oz of cooked brown rice (100 calories), 4 oz of skim milk (40 calories), 1/2 orange or 1/2 banana, soup with cooked vegetables or raw vegetables. For 1000 calories: add to the above 400 calories from a baked potato (145 calories), 4 oz of grapes or 1 apple (80–100 calories), 4 oz of fish, turkey or chicken (150 calories) and 1 slice of whole wheat bread or bran muffin (100 calories).

Update: In 1990, Robert Pritikin published *The New Pritikin Program*, essentially incorporating the principles of the original 1979 Pritikin Diet.

Caution: If you are suffering from diabetes or hypoglycemia do not use this diet without consulting your physician.

Results: "Not only is the Pritikin Diet safe and healthy, it maintains your ideal weight without any restrictions on food quantity. Unbeatable for safe, effective, long-lasting weight loss."

Our comments: A good diet if you can stick to it. For losing weight slowly, stay around 1,000 calories.

vi. The Scarsdale Medical Diet

Principle: This low calorie diet proposes a variety of fixed foods, sufficient vitamins and minerals aimed at helping people lose weight and keep it down (Tarnower and Baker, 1978). It aims at providing an average of 1,000 calories per day.

Composition: This diet is composed of proteins providing 43% of calories, fats 22.5% and carbohydrates 34.5% of the total calories. Protein sources are fish, meat, poultry, cheese and protein bread. Carbohydrates are obtained from bread, fruits and vegetables. Fats are derived from meat, eggs, cheese, poultry and nuts. Ample vitamins and minerals come from fruits, vegetables, legumes, meats, eggs and nuts.

Claims: The diet is described as safe, palatable, satisfying and uncomplicated as well as easy to prepare. It is described as nutritionally balanced, good for weight loss and adaptable in restaurants.

Basic Rules/Servings: The basic Scarsdale diet is quite rigid. It requires you to "eat exactly what is assigned" with no substitutes allowed. The diet is quite liberal in its servings of salads, fruits and vegetables. No alcohol. Carrots and celery between meals, as much as you want. Beverages to include: diet sodas, tea, and black coffee. Salads to be eaten without oil, mayonnaise, or rich dressings and vegetables without butter or margarine. Meats to be lean and poultry without skin. Stop eating when full.

Menus: These are fixed. Some of the items in the basic menu are:

Breakfast:
  1/2 grapefruit or any available fruit; 1 slice toasted protein bread; coffee/tea without sugar, milk or cream

Lunch:
  fruit salad or cold cuts; tomatoes; spinach; carrots; broccoli; 1 slice protein bread; coffee/tea

Dinner:
  fish or roast, broiled chicken or steak; salad of lettuce, tomatoes, and celery; tea/coffee

Two weeks of basic diet is followed by two weeks of keep-trim diet which requires no more than 2 slices of protein bread, no sugars, potatoes, dairy fats, candy, or desserts, but allows up to 1 1/2 oz of alcohol.

Update: The diet remained popular for a long time and even today some people use it.

Added Suggestions: The diet suggestions are supplemented with behavior modification, expending of 300 calories per day with half hour of basic exercises, using weight tables to make appropriate food choices and record keeping of weight.

Our advice: This is a fairly sensible diet, nutritionally good with vitamins and minerals and especially good if you suffer from hypoglycemia.

vii. The Jenny Craig Diet

Principle: The company provides an approach to healthy weight loss with emphasis on safety and long-term weight maintenance. This is to be achieved with a decrease in fat and increase in carbohydrate intake, moderate caloric restriction and exercise.

Composition: The menus are low in fat and cholesterol and high in complex carbohydrate and fiber. They provide 1,000 to 2,600 calories with the following composition: 60% carbohydrate; 20% protein; 20% fat; 100 mg cholesterol; 2–3 g sodium; 30 g fiber.

Claims: The Jenny Craig foods are manufactured "under strict compliance with the FDA and USDA" and are "always fresh". They contain no added MSG (monosodium glutamate) and sulfites.

Servings: The plan calls for three meals and at least three snacks to be eaten at the same times every day, no more than two to four hours apart. The servings vary with the calorie needs of the person. For instance, for a 1,200 calorie diet the servings are distributed as follows: 5 grains, 3 vegetables, 2 fruits, 6 meats, 2 milk, and 2 fats/oils. And for 1,800 calories, the servings are: 9 grains, 5 vegetables, 5 fruits, 6 meats, 2 milk, and 2 fats/oils. The plan allows flexibility in getting the number of calories appropriate for each individual. Do not miss breakfast. Drink 8 eight ounce glasses of water every day. Exercise for 30 minutes on most days. Multivitamin and mineral supplements are recommended.

Menus: Daily, weekly and vegetarian menus are available in the daily calorie levels of 1,000 to 2,300 calories. Adolescent menus are available in the calorie range of 1,500 to 2,000. For weight maintenance, the menus available are in the range of 1,200 to 2,600 calories. Also available are different weekly menus.

Ten Famous Diets: Objective Analysis and Advice 53

Update: The company communicates with physicians to seek permission to enroll their patients in this program. The program was developed by registered dietitians and the menus reflect USDA recommendations to decrease fat and increase carbohydrate in the diets.

Our comments: This is a sensible diet plan. The composition of the diet is medically sound.

viii. The Slim–Fast Diet

Principle: This diet plan replaces two meals each day with Slim–Fast shakes to lose weight. To maintain weight, one meal is replaced with a shake.

Composition: The Ultra Slim–Fast shake provides vitamins, minerals, protein and fiber. It is low in fat and packed with calcium, folic acid, niacin, and vitamins C and E. The shakes have 220 calories in a 325 ml serving with: 3 g total fat, 1 g saturated fat, 5 mg cholesterol, 220 mg sodium, 38 g carbohydrate, and 10 g protein. Two Slim–Fast shakes provide two-thirds of 18 essential vitamins and minerals.

Claims: The company claims the Slim–Fast products are nutritious, delicious in taste, convenient and easy to follow. They offer a variety of flavors and help to control calories.

Results: Three studies of over 500 people cited by the Slim–Fast Foods Company indicate that the participants using Slim–Fast lost an average of 15.6 lbs (Ditschuneit et al.), 15.2 lbs. (Haber et al., 1994), and 16.3 lbs. (Rothacker, 1998) over a twelve week period. At least 40% of the participants who were in weight maintenance program for two years kept off at least 50% of their initial weight loss.

Servings: The servings come in the form of bars and shakes. Each bar contains 120 calories and each shake has 220 calories.

Menus: The suggested typical menu is as follows

   Breakfast and Lunch:
      Slim–Fast Shake

Dinner:
> Large salad; four ounces of meat, poultry, fish or lean meat; 1/2 baked potato; 3 steamed vegetables; fruit for dessert

Snacks:
> Two pieces of fruit
> One Nutritional Energy Bar as needed

Calories: The plans provide 1,200 to 1,500 calories, 1,200 calories for small sized persons and up to 1,500 calories for larger-sized individuals.

Update: You can call the company toll–free at 1–877–SLIM–777 or visit their web site at www.slimfast.com for latest information.

Added Suggestions: The company marketing Slim–Fast products suggests that you exercise moderately to burn about 150 calories per day, keep a positive attitude and chart your weights to record success.

Our advice: This is a sensible program. Its features are its portability, good nutritional composition, and ease of use.

ix. The Weight Watcher's Diet

Principle: Born in 1963, Weight Watchers is the granddaddy of diet plans. It has helped more than 23 million people in more than 28 countries lose weight through a combination of a nutritional food program, behavior modification, exercise, and above all, support group style motivation.

Composition: Since September 1997, Weight Watchers has allowed its members to eat anything they want. That's the inspiration of their *1–2–3 Success* plan, based on the *POINTS Food System.* Here's how it works: Every food is assigned a point value based on fat, calorie and fiber content. Each member receives a daily allotment of points based on his or her body mass index (BMI), which is determined by height and weight. If you wish to "bank" points for a special occasion, you may. The only stipulations are: 1) You must fulfill the minimum requirements of nutritionally sound foods, e.g. you need to consume at least two servings of milk products per day (three for teens or adults over age fifty) and at least five

Ten Famous Diets: Objective Analysis and Advice   55

servings of fruits and vegetables. 2) You may not fall below the range of points assigned to you in order to make up for a binge.

Additional Services: Members are encouraged to attend weekly meetings that provide them with emotional support and tools to help them deal with life's ups and downs in ways that do not involve food.

Claims/Results: The *1–2–3 Success* plan is designed for weight loss of up to two pounds per week after the first three weeks. (The first weeks of the diet often represent a major loss of water weight.) Goal weight is determined by BMI of between 20 and 25 depending on age. Half of all life-time members maintain 100% of their weight loss after two years.

Servings: Servings are not weighed or measured; instead, members receive a general rule of thumb—or fist. For example, a fist equals one cup or a medium fruit, while a cupped hand equals one or two ounces of nuts or pretzels. Members must limit their intake of refined sugars and alcohol is restricted to one drink daily. They may choose one dessert two or three times a week.

Calories: The plan offers a range of 1,100 to 2,000 calorie diets.

Advice: Members are encouraged to consult a physician before embarking on the plan and are advised to take a daily vitamin pill and drink six glasses of water per day. In addition, they are expected to exercise a minimum of 20 minutes each day.

Menus:
  Breakfast:
      1/2 glass orange juice; 1 cup bran flakes; 1 cup skim milk
  Lunch:
      1 tuna salad sandwich, 1 cup aspartame sweetened yogurt with 1 slice nectarine
  Dinner:
      1 serving Southern Oven Fried Chicken (their recipe); 1 serving macaroni and cheese (their recipe); 1 serving Old Fashioned Baked Beans (their recipe); 1 cup steamed green beans; 1 cup watermelon chunks
  Snack:
      3 cups microwave popcorn

Update: In January, 1999, Weight Watcher's launched *The Daily Coach*, a series of booklets that give members skills to deal with life's challenges. These include visualization, affirmation and other behavioral techniques. (Weight Watcher's Website, 1999).

Our Comment: Weight Watcher's covers all the psychological and physical bases without locking you into a difficult eating plan. They provide recipes and menus, but you can use your own as you learn to embark on your personal healthy life choices.

x. The Nutri/System Weight Loss Program

Principle: This program meets the American Medical Association and The National Institutes of Heath standards of low–calorie meal plans, behavioral and nutritional counseling, and exercise (Schiffman and Scobey, 1990).

Composition: The menus are low in fat and cholesterol, high in complex carbohydrates, with moderate amounts of protein. The amount of fat is less than 30% of total calories, but 25% or less is considered better. The fats are divided equally among polyunsaturated, monounsaturated and saturated fats. Fifty percent of the total calories are from carbohydrates and 15–20% from proteins with 20–30 g of fiber.

Claims: Each plan is nutritionally sound. The meals are easy to prepare, calorie controlled and have intensified flavors. Each recipe lists its calorie and nutritional content.

Servings: The 1,300 calorie plan provides 8 starches, 3 low fat meats, 3 vegetables, 2 fruits, 2 low fat milks and 3 fats. The 1,500 calorie plan provides 9 starches, 3 low fat meats, 6 vegetables, 2 fruits, 2 low fat milks, and 4 fats. The 2,000 calorie plan includes 12 starches, 4 low fat meats, 6 vegetables, 3 fruits, 3 low fat milks and 5 fats.

Advice: Additional advice includes nutritional education, behavior modification and a special exercise program designed for overweight adults. The importance of exercise is stressed.

Recipes: Each recipe lists its calorie and nutritional content. There are 300 original high flavor, high texture, low calorie recipes. Fourteen days of menus are presented.

Calories: Menu plans for 1,300 calories, 1,500 calories and 2,000 calories are provided. The plans include two weeks of recipes for breakfast, lunch, dinner and snacks.

Menus: The meals can be supplemented with unlimited quantities of lettuce, celery, cucumber, parsley, radishes, club soda, seltzer, mineral water, diet sodas, decaffeinated tea or coffee. A typical menu resembles:

Breakfast:
  yogurt; fruit; slice of whole wheat toast with 1 tsp margarine; skim milk; tea or coffee
Snack:
  English muffin
Lunch:
  tomato soup; beef teriyaki; brown rice
Snack:
  fruit or cookie
Dinner:
  chicken paprikash; noodles; vegetable; 1 teaspoon margarine; skim milk; tea or coffee

Update: Nutri/System was founded in 1971. In 1987 products with intensified flavor were added. The company has over 1,500 weight loss centers in North America.

Our comment: For weight control this is one of the sensible plans especially if combined with behavior modification, nutritional counseling and exercise.

References

American Dietetic Association (1997). Website: http://www.eatright.org.

American Heart Association. (1998). *Step I and Step II Diets.* Website: http//www.americanheart.org.

Ditschuneit, H.W., et al. Metabolic and weight loss effects on long–term dietary intervention in obese patients. *American Journal of Clinical Nutrition.* (in press).

Herber, D., et al. (1994). Clinical evaluation of a minimal intervention meal replacement regimen for weight reduction. *Journal of American College of Nutrition, 13,* 605–14.

Lindsay, A. (1998). *The American Cancer Society Cookbook.* NY, NY: Heart Books.

Ornish, D. (1990). *Dr. Dean Ornish's Program for Reversing Heart Disease.* New York, NY: Ballantine Books.

Ornish, D. et al. (1998). Intensive lifestyle changes for reversal of coronary heart disease. *Journal of the American Medical Association, 280,* 2001–2007.

Pritikin, N. and McGrady, P.M. (1997). *The Pritikin Program for Diet and Exercise.* New York, NY: Grosset and Dunlap.

Rothacker, D. (1998). Five–year weight control with meal replacements: Comparison with background in rural Wisconsin. *International Journal of Obesity, 22,* 256S.

Schiffman, S.S. and Scobey, J. (1990). *The NutriSystem Flavor Set–Point Weight Loss Cookbook.* Boston MA: Little, Brown and Co.

Tarnower, H. and Baker, S. (1978). *The Complete Scarsdale Medical Diet.* New York, NY: Dawson, Wade Publishers, Inc.

United States Department of Agriculture. (1997). *The Food Guide Pyramid.* Website: http://www.usda.gov.

Weight Watcher's. (1999). Website: http://www.weightwatchers.com.

Chapter 6

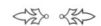

❧ ❧

International Restaurants: How to Eat Healthy at Each

Let's eat out tonight. We will be your restaurant guides through this chapter, watching your health at all times.

The National Restaurant Association estimates that nearly half of all Americans eat out every day! Dual careers, single parenting, business meetings and overwork are some of the factors accounting for large numbers of people eating out. You are probably not an exception.

So, what is in this chapter for you? The most commonly frequented international restaurants have been selected for discussion. We will provide guidance for you as we visit each of them. You will discover how to enjoy your favorite foods in a healthful way. You will be advised on how to make well-informed food selections and you will learn to personalize the calculations of your calorie and fat budget. Here you will find every principle of good nutrition and healthy eating. Following the general information, there will be specifics on ordering at each of the ten types of restaurants. The type of cooking, items to order and to avoid will be identified. A complete healthy menu will be provided for each restaurant. To round out the information, the calorie count of the menu and the amount of total fat, saturated fat, cholesterol and sodium will be presented. [For more information, refer to Warshaw (1990) and Lichten (1998).]

For a joyous evening, with the mission in mind to improve your health and promote longevity, let us set the stage to explore the art and science of eating out. First, develop a healthy mindset and plan ahead. Remember that 40% of restaurant customers try to eat healthy, be one them. Also remember that 40% of restaurants feature healthy menu items (Lichten, 1998). In the rest of them, you will need to coach the waiter to create what you want.

Exercise care in selecting a restaurant. Opt for a quiet, not too noisy one. Make a reservation to avoid standing in line. If you know the restaurant, reserve seats with a good vantage point and the right atmosphere. Keep ample time for the meal. Your dining experience should be a relaxed, tension free excursion. Enjoy the company, appreciate the environment, and compliment the waiter. Make dining out a pleasurable event, not a binge-eating event.

Avoid buffet places; there will be too many saboteurs and it will be hard to resist some of them. Shun all-you-can-eat places because you would want to eat more than what you paid for. Preserve the principles of proper eating, particularly at parties and picnics. You will find a lot of seducers there. Be aware of the dangers of eating out—too many calories, too much fat, too much salt, and the resulting regrets.

Once you have decided on a restaurant, think about the ordering. First, pay attention to the healthy menu items earmarked by the restaurants as good for you. If your weight is the main concern, determine the number of calories you are entitled to for the meal you are going to have in the restaurant. Complete calorie counts are in the tables elsewhere, but remember the following few:

Coca Cola/Pepsi (12 oz)	140 calories
Red wine (5 oz)	107 calories
Bread (1 slice)	70 calories
Butter (1 Tbl)	100 calories
Small side salad	25–30 calories
Baked potato (4 oz)	124 calories
Red salmon (6 oz)	280 calories
Sirloin steak (6 oz)	220 calories
Ice cream (2 oz)	120 calories
Cheesecake (2 oz)	220 calories

To protect your heart, let us remind you, the daily calorie intake from fats should be 30% or less of the total and the cholesterol intake should be less than 300 mg per day. Therefore, to make your meal heart-healthy, order foods that are low in total fat, saturated fatty acids and cholesterol. Request a cooking method with less fat and select foods that are baked, broiled or boiled rather than fried. Choose foods that are low in sodium or special order to meet your needs. Request serving of the sauces, condiments and seasonings on the side so you can decide how much of each of those you should use. Do not hesitate to say no MSG. Practice portion control or make a meal out of an appetizer. Here are the eleven types of restaurants we are going to visit:

i. Chinatown Chinese Restaurant

Ten Tips and Facts:

1. Chinese food is high in sodium. Order preparations with instructions to serve low sodium.
2. Choose white rice; avoid fried rice.
3. Avoid fried, breaded and fried, coated and crispy preparations.
4. Lo Mein noodles are good and healthy. Order low fat, low sodium.
5. Avoid deep fried pork, beef, chicken, spare ribs, and egg rolls. All are high in fat and sodium.
6. Avoid sweet and sour preparations with nuts.
7. Instead of high fat appetizers choose low sodium rice soup, Chinese vegetable soup or chicken soup.
8. For proteins pick chicken, tofu (bean curd), shrimp, scallops and fish. Choose preparations with green beans and broccoli.
9. For dessert pick pineapple or lychee. Avoid ice cream.
10. Take a fortune cookie, read the fortune and leave the cookie.

Healthy Choices on a Chinese Menu:

Appetizers: Steamed Peking Ravioli; Teriyaki chicken
Soups: Wonton; Rice and Chicken Soup; Vegetable, chicken, or Beef Strips Soup

Entrées: Velvet chicken; Hunan Spicy Chicken; Shrimp or Beef with Broccoli; Fresh Fish Fillets; Beef Chow Mein
Desserts: Pineapple chunks; Lychee pieces; Ice cream

Healthy Chinese Menu

Analysis of Menu

Hot and sour soup
Yu-hsiang chicken
Shrimp with broccoli
Steamed white rice
Pineapple chunks

Total calories: 650
32% as fat
28% as protein
40% as carbohydrates
15 mg as cholesterol
1,200 mg as sodium

ii. Great American Steakhouse

Ten Tips and Facts:

1. Expect the food to be made to your order.
2. Instruct the waiter that you want the beef broiled or grilled without additional fat or salt.
3. Choose a lean cut like filet mignon or London broil.
4. Go for a small portion, 6 oz.
5. Advise the waiter that the visible fat be trimmed before broiling.
6. When the steak is served, trim off any visible fat before eating.
7. Order green salad with dressing on the side.
8. Choose fresh steamed vegetables and a baked potato with a small amount of margarine or low-fat yogurt.
9. Select low-calorie clear soup.
10. Enjoy a glass of red wine.

Healthy Choices on a Steakhouse Menu

Appetizers: Mixture of fresh fruit
Soups: Clear soup or cream of chicken soup
Salads: Green leafy vegetables

Entrées: Filet mignon, 6 oz with baked potato
Desserts: Cheese cake

Healthy Steakhouse Menu	**Analysis of Menu**
Small house salad or Caesar salad: dressing on side	Total Calories: 650
	28% as fat
Clear soup with vegetables	28% as protein
Filet mignon – 6 oz (broiled)	44% as carbohydrates
Baked potato w/ low-fat yogurt	180 mg cholesterol
broccoli, tomato, vegetable	900 mg sodium
Glass of red wine	
Coffee	

iii. American Restaurant

Ten Tips and Facts:

1. Salads with turkey or chicken with dressing on the side.
2. Order baked potato instead of French fries.
3. Good appetizer—peel-and-eat shrimp or bowl of chili.
4. Soup must be low sodium.
5. House salad or Cobb salad with vegetables but without cheese, bacon and egg.
6. Avoid melts, cheese steaks (sandwich).
7. Avoid soft drinks—drink water.
8. Best dessert—fruit.
9. Avoid all-fat dips with shrimp or raw bar selections.
10. Order sandwich on whole-wheat bread.

Healthy Choices on an American Menu:

Appetizer: Peel-and-eat shrimp; chili (without cheese); vegetable gumbo (vegetables, onions, tomatoes, broccoli, green beans simmered in Cajun spices)

Salad: House salad or blackened chicken salad

Sandwich: Blackened chicken sandwich
Burger: Veggie Burger (sautéed onions, peppers, mushrooms)
Hot entrée: Teriyaki chicken breast.
Side Orders: Rice pilaf, baked potato.
Dessert: Sorbet (lemon or raspberry)

Healthy American Menu

Analysis of Menu

Peel-and-eat shrimp
Chili (without cheese)
Baked potato
Teriyaki chicken breast
Sorbet

Total calories: 800
22% as fat
25% protein
53% as carbohydrates
160 mg cholesterol
1,000 mg sodium

iv. Seafood Gourmet

Ten Tips and Facts:

1. Seafood is the healthiest protein food. It is good for those with heart disease, high blood pressure and weight problems.
2. Seafood is low in calories, saturated fat and moderately high in cholesterol.
3. Fish have high fish oils (Omega-3 fats) which are polyunsaturated fats. They lower triglycerides.
4. Shellfish is low in saturated fats and low in sodium.
5. Surimi, a crabmeat look alike, is low in calories, fat and cholesterol but high in sodium.
6. For low calorie, low fat items go to the raw bar for raw oysters, clams, sushi and sashimi.
7. Avoid buttered preparations
8. Remember shrimp is very high in cholesterol (166 mg in 3 oz).
9. Order Cajun style cooking.
10. A good appetizer: boiled cocktail shrimp.

Healthy Choices on a Seafood Gourmet Menu

Raw bar:	Oysters on the half-shell
Appetizers:	Barbecued Shrimp; Marinated Calamari
Soups:	Shrimp gumbo, Clam Chowder
Entrées:	Mahi Mahi (dolphin), Salmon, Surimi, Boiled Maine Lobster w/lemon, Alaskan King Crab, Scallops w/ Spicy Tomato, Baked Potato, Steamed Broccoli, Saffron Rice
Desserts:	Watermelon, Strawberries with Cream

Healthy Seafood Menu

Tossed green salad
Clam chowder soup
Two vegetables
Sautéed scallops in tomato sauce
Mahi Mahi Cajun style
Rice pilaf
Coffee

Analysis of Menu

Total calories 800
20% as fat
30% as protein
50% as carbohydrate
180 mg cholesterol
800 mg as sodium

v. A Night Out in Italy

Ten Tips and Facts:

1. Go for a cup of soup: minestrone or stacciatalla.
2. Make a good salad with arugula, broccoli, beets, onions, peppers, raw vegetables, spinach and tomatoes.
3. Garlic bread is all right but not soaked with olive oil. You will end up with too much fat and too many calories.
4. A little bit of olive oil is acceptable. It is a monounsaturated fat that lowers cholesterol.
5. Avoid crusty bread with creamy butter.
6. Squid, clam or mussels are good constituents of a healthy antipasto.

7. For a healthy pasta choose marinara, primavera, white clam sauce, tomato and basil.
8. If you can afford an extra 10% in calories, a glass of red wine will please your palate.
9. Avoid the selection of large, creamy, nutty desserts. Opt for an Italian ice.
10. Relax with demitasse of espresso.

Healthy Choices on an Italian Menu

Antipasto:	Marinated calamari or mushrooms, steamed clams in white wine
Soup:	Tortellini in broth
Salad:	House salad
Pasta:	Angel hair or Ziti Bolognese
Meat:	Veal cacciatore or chicken primavera.
Fish:	Shrimp primavera or marinara or sole primavera
Dessert:	Italian Ice

Healthy Italian Menu	**Analysis of Menu:**
Arugula and belgian endive salad	Total calories 700
Fusilli pasta with no sauce	20% as fat
Shrimp primavera	30% as protein
Red wine	50% as carbohydrate
Italian ice	165 mg cholesterol
Espresso	700 mg sodium

vi. A Meal in the Middle East

Ten Tips and Facts:

1. Avoid fried foods and egg preparations; they are high in cholesterol.
2. Avoid the dessert, Baklava, very high in calories and fat.

3. Pita—flat round bread, and rice pilaf are common healthy items.
4. Tabouli—cold cracked wheat, a healthy item.
5. Vegetables—commonly served are eggplants, onions, and tomatoes in salads.
6. Shish kabob with chicken marinated in lemon, grilled on a skewer with vegetables. Great entrée. Take it without olives, which are high in sodium.
7. Try a stuffed dish with cabbage or eggplant as an alternative to shish kabobs.
8. Rarely serve seafood. You may not get alcoholic drinks in some restaurants.
9. Take yogurt as a side order.
10. Food is generally healthy in middle eastern cuisines.

Healthy Choices on a Middle Eastern Menu

Appetizers:	Dolma (hot grape leaves stuffed with spicy ground lamb, rice and onions); Ful Medames
Soups:	Green vegetable soup with lemon; Mushroom soup; Chickpea and lentil soup; Chicken broth
Side orders:	Tabouli; rice pilaf; steamed vegetables; pita bread
Entrées:	Shish kabob; Stuffed cabbage or eggplant
Dessert:	Rice pudding; Sponge cake; Minted tea; Turkish coffee

Healthy Middle Eastern Menu	**Analysis of Menu**
Tabouli salad	Total calories 700
Pita bread	30% as fat
Rice pilaf	25% as protein
Chicken shish kabob	45% as carbohydrates
Turkish coffee	170 mg cholesterol
	900 mg sodium

vii. The Mexican Treat

Ten Tips and Facts:

1. Most items are high in sodium. Special order low sodium preparations.
2. Avoid items with sour cream, guacamole, and cheese.
3. Avoid fried or deep fried items.
4. Corn, chili and beans are good carbohydrate-rich items.
5. Red or green salsa made with tomatoes, onions and spices is good but high in sodium.
6. Go easy on chips.
7. Black bean soup is nutritionally good.
8. Avoid fried tortilla chips with cheese (super nachos).
9. A low sodium Mexican dinner salad is good. Use salsa as salad dressing.
10. Daiquiris go well with Mexican food.

Healthy Choices on a Mexican Menu

Appetizers:	Chips; nachos; soft tacos
Soups:	Black bean soup; Chili con carne without cheese; Gazpacho; Ceviche
Side orders:	Black beans; Mexican rice; Soft flour tortillas with beans
Entrées:	Chicken or beef enchiladas; Burritos; Fajitas; Mexican Salad with spicy chicken
Dessert:	Flan (custard)

Healthy Mexican Menu

Black bean soup
Chili con carne
Salsa
Vegetables
Dinner salad with chicken
Soft taco
Daiquiri

Analysis of Menu

Total calories 650
30% as fat
25% as protein
45% as carbohydrates
100 mg cholesterol
1,200 mg sodium

Ten International Restaurants: How to Eat Healthy at Each   69

viii. The Japanese Restaurant

Ten Tips and Facts:

1. Generally clean and hygienic.
2. Healthiest food in the world.
3. Less fat than in other international restaurants.
4. The cooking oils employed are generally very low in cholesterol.
5. Generally too much sodium; order sashimi, steamed rice, salad to lower amount of sodium. Put sauces on side.
6. Foods usually boiled, broiled, steamed and braised.
7. Sushi, sashimi (raw fish)—safe? Yes.
8. Avoid fried foods.
9. You get protein from tofu-soy bean curd. This is used in entrees, soups and salads.
10. A surprise—soup will be served at the end of the meal.

Healthy Choices on a Japanese Menu:

Starter: Sashimi tuna or salmon; sashimi combination of tuna, salmon or lobster; sushi combination.
Appetizer: Yutofu (hot bean curd); Shumai (steamed shrimp).
Soup: Suimono (clear broth soup); Yaki-udon (noodle soup)
Salads: Tossed salad; Tofu salad; Seafood salad
Entrées: Teriyaki chicken, salmon, beef or seafood combination; Sukiyaki chicken (sliced chicken with vegetables); Shabu-shabu (sliced beef with vegetables)
Dessert: Fresh fruit

Healthy Japanese Menu

Sashimi Tuna
Yaki-udon soup
Steamed rice
Tofu salad
Fresh fruit

Analysis of Menu

Total calories 600
15% as fat
30% as protein
55% as carbohydrates
80 mg cholesterol
1,400 sodium

ix. Cafe de Paris

Ten Tips and Facts:

1. "Wine is a professor of taste. By teaching us inner awareness, wine liberates the mind and enlightens the spirit." – Paul Clauder. Know your wines before you go to a French restaurant.
2. Grilled marinated shrimp is a good appetizer.
3. Order clear soup with vegetables. Avoid creamy soups. If you order French onion soup, order low sodium and take out cheese.
4. Green salads are great. Order without bacon and eggs.
5. For proteins order fish or chicken which have less cholesterol, fat and saturated fat. Avoid duck.
6. For carbohydrates pick baked potato, brown rice or rice pilaf.
7. Avoid bread, butter, cheese sauce, and sausage.
8. Fruits will make a great dessert.
9. Liquor has calories but not fat or cholesterol.
10. Advise the waiter to use healthy cooking method—Cajun, grilled, poached or stir-fried.

Healthy Choices on a French Menu

Appetizer:	Vegetable meringue with mustard sauce.
Soup:	French onion soup.
Salad:	House salad with lettuce, onions, peppers and sprouts.
Entrées:	Petite filet mignon or chicken sautéed (with tomatoes, herbs, and asparagus in olive oil) or poached salmon with smoked tomato sauce and cilantro.
Vegetable:	Snow peas sautéed with red pepper.
Desserts:	Fresh strawberries topped with Chambord liquor.

Healthy French Menu

French onion soup
    low salt (no cheese)
Salad with exotic greens
    (dressing on side)

Analysis of Menu

Total calories 800
30% as fat
20% as protein
50% as carbohydrates

Healthy French Menu *cont.*

Poached Salmon
    or filet mignon (6 oz)
Baked potato with cream
Strawberries without cream
    Red wine, 6 oz

Analysis of Menu *cont.*

200 mg cholesterol
850 mg sodium

x. The Taj Majal: An Indian Cuisine

Ten Tips and Facts:

1. Lentil soup is the best, order low sodium.
2. For special bread, order Chappati or Nan, but without butter or oil.
3. Order stewed, boiled or steamed items.
4. Rice is the main part of a meal. Ask for Basmati rice. It has excellent flavor.
5. Tandoori chicken without skin is tasty and healthy. Go for it, it is good for protein, low in cholesterol and calories.
6. Avoid pork, lamb and beef.
7. For fiber and non-meat protein choose vegetables, chickpeas and lentils.
8. Avoid items cooked in coconut milk, which is rich in calories and saturated fat, and avoid ghee (Indian butter).
9. Majority of restaurants are poor in seafood. Don't expect fresh seafood.
10. For a complete vegetarian dinner order "Thali" which is a combination of rice, bread (chappati, puree or nan), vegetables, papadam (wafer) and raita (a mixture of cut cucumbers, onions and yogurt).

Healthy Choices on an Indian Menu

Appetizers:	Papadam; vegetable samosa (peas and potatoes wrapped in fried crust)
Soup:	Lentil soup
Salad:	Rarely served; raita is the substitute

Vegetables:	Curry made with peas, potatoes, and tomatoes; Vegetable pilaf (rice and vegetables)
Non-vegetarian items:	Chicken tikka; Tandoori chicken; chicken, beef or shrimp curry or biryani
Meal accompaniment:	Raita
Dessert:	Mango Kulfi; Kheer (rice pudding); Gulab jamun (warm balls of donut-like round dough fried in honey sauce)

Healthy Indian Menu

Lentil soup (8 oz)
Papadam
Nan or Chappati
Vegetable curry
Steamed rice
Chicken Tandoori
   or chicken tikka
Raita

Analysis of Menu:

Total calories 600
22% as fat
23% as protein
55% as carbohydrate
130 mg cholesterol
800 mg sodium

xi. The Thai Restaurant

Ten Tips and Facts:

1. Thai cooking uses coconut oil or lard. Very high in saturated fat.
2. Curries have a lot of coconut oil; eat sparingly.
3. Avoid deep fried, stir-fried, crispy items.
4. Avoid high fat drinks.
5. Avoid fried chicken wings. They are high in calories, fat and sodium.
6. Steamed mussels are all right.
7. Healthy soup is Tom Yum Koong.
8. Go for garden salad.
9. Steamed rice is fine.
10. Choose chicken, shrimp or fish with vegetables as an entrée. Ask for low sodium preparations.

Healthy Choices on a Thai Menu

Appetizers: Steamed mussels; chicken or beef satay; seafood kabob
Soups: Tom Yum Koong (shrimp soup); crystal noodle—clear soup with chicken, bean, noodles and vegetables
Salad: Green mixed garden salad with tofu
Curry: Green, red or yellow (cooked in coconut milk); Thai chicken sautéed with cashews, onions, mushrooms and chili; Beef basil sautéed with hot basil leaves; Seafood combination; Vegetables; Rice; Noodles
Desserts: Lychee nuts; Fried bananas; Thai custard

Healthy Thai Menu	Analysis of Menu
Tom Yum Koong	Total calories 625
Steamed rice	30% as fat
Thai chicken	20% as protein
Seafood combination (Poy Sian)	50% as carbohydrates
Fried banana	160 mg cholesterol
Mineral water	1,200 mg sodium

References

Lichten, J.V. (1998). *Driving Lean. How to Eat Healthy in Your Favorite Restaurants.* Houston, TX: Nutrifit Publishing.

Warshaw, H.S. (1990). *The Restaurant Companion: A Guide to Healthier Eating Out.* New York: Surrey Books.

Chapter 7

Ten Fast Foods: Yes, They Are OK

Fast food is commonly described as "junk" food. This is a misnomer. Surprisingly, many nutritious and healthy items can be found at fast food places.

It is important to develop a sensible mind set and avoid the many costly temptations. If you are going to frequent these places you should remember the basic facts about total fat, saturated fat, cholesterol and sodium. If you have medical problems like coronary artery disease, high cholesterol, high blood pressure or diabetes, it is important to be aware of the nutritional value of items at fast food places. This chapter presents some reasons why so many Americans eat at these places and submits a list of ten general tips on fast food eating. This is followed by an analysis of the nutritional value of the most commonly ordered meals at each of the largest fast food chains. The constituents of these items are detailed with a special focus on calories, total fat, saturated fat, cholesterol and sodium. "Best choices" from each chain are identified and a "Healthy meal" recommendation with calorie counts presented. The reader is advised to refer to two excellent sources for more detailed information (Franz, 1998; Jacobson and Fritschner, 1991).

Ten Reasons Why We Eat at Fast Food Places

1. To save time: This is probably the biggest reason. Since we are too busy working, we have no time to cook, relax and eat.
2. Convenient locations. The chances are that any one of the fast food places is closer to home or work than regular restaurants.

3. Fast service: We are an "On the Go" society. We just want "pay and pick in a minute" service. Fast food places provide that.
4. Variety of choices: Fast food places have many items that appeal to adults and children. It is much more convenient to feed children in a chain restaurant than in a sit-down restaurant.
5. Open for breakfast, lunch and dinner: We don't have patience to cook breakfast at home or take an hour away from work for lunch and we are too tired or busy for a proper dinner. For any time of day fast food is there.
6. No tipping: Fast foods are relatively inexpensive and no tipping is an added attraction.
7. No dress code: You can walk into any fast food place in your uniform, soiled work clothes or fancy suits without having to worry about any criticism.
8. Drive through pick-ups: Most fast food places have these for added convenience and quicker service.
9. They are open late, often until 11 pm or midnight, convenient for that late night snack.
10. Power of advertisements: Children's happy meals with toys, two-for-the-price-of-one offers and free drinks are some of the ways the consumer is impacted and attracted to fast food restaurants.

Ten Tips on Fast Food Eating

1. Eat fast food slowly. Fast food doesn't have to be eaten on the run.
2. Sensible eating means being aware of basic facts about your body's needs. Know your daily calorie requirements and the limits of intake of total fat, saturated fat, cholesterol and sodium good for you.
3. Eat the right way. Take small bites, chew the food completely before swallowing and do not take the next bite before you swallow the last morsel.
4. Cut down on soda and shakes, instead drink iced tea, fruit juice or skim milk. Never hesitate to ask for water.
5. To reduce sodium intake, order french fries without added salt, and go easy on ketchup and barbecue sauce.

6. Avoid breaded and deep-fried fish and chicken sandwiches, which may be loaded with saturated fat.
7. Remove all skin and crusts from fried chicken preparations.
8. Don't get swayed to order a larger meal than you want by the "value meals" which may be less money for more food.
9. Limit the number of times you eat fast food per week, save it for "emergency situations".
10. To make your own healthy meal, look for a salad bar. Enjoy salad with vegetables, Italian or French dressing and whole-grain bread.

Now, let us look at some popular fast food restaurant meals. If you are health-conscious or your health requires restrictions pay special attention to the "Best choices" and "Healthy meal" suggested for each of the places discussed here.

McDonald's

The Meal

Big Mac:
    weight 215 g   calories 500   protein 25 g
    carbohydrates 42 g   added sugar 5 g   fat 26 g
    % calories from fat 47 saturated fat 9 g   sodium 890 mg
    cholesterol 100 mg

Coca Cola–12 oz:
    weight 360 g   calories 140   protein 0 g
    carbohydrates 38 g   added sugar 38 g   sodium 15 mg

French Fries–medium:
    weight 97 g   calories 320   protein 4 g
    carbohydrates 36 g   fat 17 g   % calories from fat 48
    saturated fat 4 g   sodium 150 g   Iron % U.S. RDA 4
    Vitamin C % U.S. RDA 20

Meal Total: 960 calories, 100 mg cholesterol, 1,055 mg sodium, and 47–48 % calories from fat

Ten Fast Foods: Yes, They Are OK

Analysis of the Meal

Too much fat—not good for heart patients (should be less than 30% calories from fat). Calorie count is too high if you are on a low calorie diet or trying to lose weight. Sodium amount is high at 1,055 mg (persons with high blood pressure should limit sodium intake to less than 1,000 mg per day). Cholesterol is one-third of whole day's total.

Best healthy choices at McDonald's: Regular hamburger or McLean Deluxe.

Healthy meal at McDonald's: regular hamburger (255 calories), side salad (30 calories), low fat milk (1% fat) or orange juice:

Burger King

The Meal

Whopper:
    weight 270 g   calories 614   protein 27 g
    carbohydrates 45 g   fat 36 g   saturated fat 12 g
    % calories from fat 53 cholesterol 90 mg sodium 865 mg

Coca Cola–13 oz: calories 156

French Fries–medium: calories 372

Meal Total: 1,142 calories, 48-53 % calories from fat, 1,118 mg sodium

Analysis of the Meal

High fat content not good for the heart. Too many calories in one meal out of three. Sodium content too high for hypertension. Cholesterol is almost one-third of total recommended daily intake.

Best choice at Burger King: BK Broiler chicken sandwich.

Healthy meal at Burger King: BK Broiler chicken sandwich (267 calories), side salad (25 calories), orange juice, (182 calories): Total calories 374.

Kentucky Fried Chicken (KFC)

The Meal

Original Recipe 2 pieces–breast and thigh:
   weight 473 g   calories 1,002   protein 55 g
   carbohydrates 73 g   fat 55 g   saturated fat 14 g
   % calories from fat 49   cholesterol 222 mg   sodium 2,482 mg

Pepsi: calories 140

Meal Total: 1,142 calories, 49% calories from fat, 2467 mg sodium

Analysis of the Meal

High calorie meal. Fat content too high. Cholesterol level unacceptable. Sodium content too high even for healthy people. Not good for heart, high blood pressure or obesity. Eat only after removing all skin.

Best healthy choice at KFC: Extra crispy two thighs (discard skin).

Healthy meal at KFC: Two extra crispy thighs minus skin (400 calories), corn (176 calories), baked beans (133 calories): Total calories 709.

Pizza Hut

The Meal

Pan Pizza, supreme, 2 slices:
   weight 255 g   calories 589   protein 32 g
   carbohydrates 53 g   fat 30 g   saturated fat 14 g
   % calories from fat 46   cholesterol 48 mg   sodium 1,363

Pepsi: calories 140

Meal Total: 729 calories, 46% calories from fat, 1378 mg sodium

Analysis of Meal

Calories slightly high. Percentage of calories from fat undesirably high. Cholesterol okay. Sodium content high. Fat content high (maybe eat only one slice). Order thin extra crispy pizza with less cheese.

Best choice at Pizza Hut: All-you-can-eat salad.

Healthy meal at Pizza Hut: Thin'n crispy, thin, medium, 2 slices (398 calories), All-you-can-eat salad.

Hardee's

The Meal

Quarter pound cheeseburger:
    weight 182 g   calories 500   protein 29 g
carbohydrates 34   fat 29 g   saturated fat 14 g
    % calories from fat 52   cholesterol 70 mg   sodium 1,060 mg

French fries–4 oz: calories 360

Coca Cola or Pepsi: calories 140

Meal Total: 1,000 calories, 52% calories from fat, 1075 mg sodium.

Analysis of the Meal

High calorie meal. Fat content not good for heart. Percentage of calories from fat too high. Sodium content high.

Best healthy choices at Hardee's: Real Lean Deluxe, grilled chicken sandwich or hamburger.

Healthy meal at Hardee's: Grilled chicken sandwich (310 calories), regular fries, and orange juice, total calories 620.

Wendy's

The Meal

Big Classic:
    weight 260 g   calories 640   protein 31 g
    carbohydrates 47 g   fat 33 mg   saturated fat 6 g
    % calories from fat 52   cholesterol 90 mg   sodium 1,085 mg

French fries (small)–3.2 oz. calories 240

Coca Cola–12 oz. calories 156

Meal Total: 1,036 calories, 48–52% calories from fat, 1250 mg sodium

Analysis of the Meal

Too many calories in one meal. High fat content. High sodium content. Percentage of calories from fat high.

Best heatlhy choices at Wendy's: Grilled chicken sandwich, Junior Hamburger

Healthy meal at Wendy's: Baked potato, garden salad with reduced calorie Italian dressing, low fat milk, Total calories 550.

Domino's Pizza

The Meal

Cheese Pizza, 2 slices, 16" thick crust.
   calories 376   protein 22 g   carbohydrates 56 g
   fat 10 g   % calories from fat 24   saturated fat 5 g
   cholesterol 19 mg   sodium 483 mg

Coca Cola–12 oz. calories 140

Meal Total: 516 calories, 24% calories from fat, 498 mg sodium

Analysis of the Meal

Calorie count is good. Fat content is acceptable. Percentage of calories from fat satisfactory. Cholesterol level excellent. Sodium content good.

Best healthy choice at Domino's: Cheese pizza, two slices (16" thin crust)

Healthy meal at Domino's Pizza: Cheese pizza, 2 slices (16" thin crust) with tomato sauce; topped pizza with mushrooms and green pepper; Water or iced tea: Total calories 620.

Taco Bell

The Meal

Two beef tacos, hard shell:
- weight 156 g calories 366 protein 20 g
- carbohydrates 22 g fat 22 g saturated fat 10 g
- % calories from fat 54 cholesterol 64 mg sodium 552 mg.

Pepsi: calories 140

Meal Total: 506 calories, 54% calories from fat, 537 mg sodium

Analysis of the Meal

Calorie count is good. Fat content high. Percentage of calories from fat not good. Cholesterol okay. Sodium content high. Overall not too bad.

Best healthy choices at Taco Bell: Soft chicken taco or chicken burrito, no red sauce.

Healthy meal from Taco Bell: Soft chicken taco (213 calories), chicken salad (125 calories), and water. Total calories: 338.

Dairy Queen

The Meal

Double hamburger with cheese:
- weight 226 g calories 570 protein 37 g
- carbohydrates 35 g fat 34 g saturated fat 18 g
- % calories from fat 54 cholesterol 120 mg sodium 1,070 mg

Coca Cola: calories 140

Meal Total: 710 calories, 54% calories from fat, 1,085 mg sodium

Analysis of the Meal

Calories high. Total fat content high. Percentage of calories from fat very high. Saturated fat high. Cholesterol high. Sodium content high.

Best healthy choices at Dairy Queen: Grilled chicken fillet sandwich, BBQ Beef sandwich.

Healthy meal at Dairy Queen: Grilled chicken fillet sandwich, salad with tomato, lettuce and onion from salad bar, banana and water to drink.

Arby's

The Meal

Roast Beef Giant:
weight 227 g	calories 530	protein 36 g
carbohydrates 41 g	fat 27 g	saturated fat 10 g
% calories from fat 46	cholesterol 78 mg	sodium 908 mg

French fries–medium: calories 394

Coca Cola–12 oz: calories 140

Meal Total: 1,064 calories, 46–48% calories from fat, 1073 mg sodium

Analysis of the Meal

Total calories high. Percentage of calories from fat high. Sodium high.

Best healthy choices at Arby's: Light Roast Chicken Deluxe (253 calories); Light Roast Beef Deluxe (296 calories).

Healthy meal at Arby's: Light Roast Beef Deluxe (296 calories), side salad (25 calories), 2% milk, 8 oz. (121 calories). Total calories: 442.

References

Franz, M.J. (1991). *Fast Food Facts*. Minneapolis, MN: IDC Publishing.

Jacobson, M.F. (1991). *Fast Food Guide*. New York, NY: Workman Publishing.

Chapter 8

Food as Medicine: Diet Prescriptions

Introduction

Food is the most important environmental factor that can tip the health odds in a person's favor or tilt them against him. Good nutrition is known to reduce the risk of a host of diseases such as diabetes, heart disease, hypertension, osteoporosis, and cancer. Many of these conditions are familial. However, what you do or don't eat can make a big difference. Often all you need to do is make a small change in your diet.

In the past we have invented several medical diets. In this chapter we combine our experiences and the wisdom of major medical organizations to formulate several target menus. Ten common conditions are targeted for prevention and treatment with diet. This discussion is aimed at presenting principles, general guidance and specifics (for 1,500 and 2,000 calorie intakes). Food is medicine and these prescriptions are your longevity diets specifically designed for the following conditions: Heart Disease, Cancer, Diabetes, Hypoglycemia, Gout, Hypertension, and Ulcers.

i. For a Healthy Individual

This diet is heart-healthy. It is essentially the same as the Step I diet described in Chapter 6. The only difference is that, for a healthy individual, the use of it does not have to be medically supervised.

Menus

1,500 Calories

Breakfast
1 grapefruit
1 cup cornflakes
1 cup 1 % milk
1 cup fresh strawberries

Lunch
Corn on the cob (6 inch)
1 tsp. margarine
2 oz boiled chicken thigh
1 pear
Tossed salad w/ tomato & cucumber
3 graham crackers

Dinner
4 oz sirloin steaks, broiled with 1 Tbl. steak sauce
1 baked potato with 1 tsp. margarine
2 oz low fat, low salt, cheddar cheese
1 cup fresh fruit salad
1/2 cup streamed squash
1/2 cup frozen yogurt

2,000 Calories

Breakfast
2 egg whites
1 bagel
1-2 tsp. margarine, unsalted
1 cup 1 % milk
1/2 cup orange juice

Lunch
2 slices of roast beef
2 slices of whole wheat toast
2 tsp. mayonnaise
1 leaf lettuce w/1 slice tomato
1/2 cup cranberry juice
1/2 cup frozen yogurt

Dinner
1 small hamburger patty with 1 hamburger bun
1 tsp. ketchup
1 leaf lettuce
1 oz part skim mozzarella cheese
1 corn on the cob
4 oatmeal raisin cookies

ii. Heart Healthy Menu

This diet is for the treatment of high cholesterol. It is the step II diet discussed in Chapter 6. (American Heart Association Website, 1996). It is to be used in conjunction with the Step I diet under medical supervision.

Menus

1,500 Calories

Breakfast
1 cup blueberries
1 cup plain low fat yogurt
1 cup cornflakes
1 cup 1% milk
1 slice whole wheat toast

Lunch
3 oz processed turkey
2 tsps. mayonnaise
2 slices of tomato
1 leaf of lettuce
2 slices whole wheat bread
1 pear or 1 cup fresh grapes

Dinner
8 oz grilled chicken
1/2 cup green peas
1 tsp. margarine
1 cup steamed carrots

1 cup tossed salad with
1/2 cup grated carrots with vinegar
1 1/2 cup fresh strawberries

2,000 Calories

Breakfast
1/2 cup fruit juice
1 medium bagel
1 cup skim milk
1 tsp. margarine
1 egg

Lunch
2 thin slices of roast beef
2 tsps. mayonnaise
2 slices of tomato
1 leaf of lettuce
2 slices whole wheat bread
8 crackers
Tossed salad: 1 cup lettuce,
1 tomato, unsalted french dressing
1 cup frozen yogurt

Dinner
4 oz broiled salmon
1/2 cup new potatoes with parsley and 1 tsp margarine
1/2 cup corn with 1 tsp. margarine
1 dinner roll
1/2 steamed broccoli
1 frosted cupcake

iii. Anti-Cancer Diet

The principle of anti-cancer diets is to include items rich in antioxidants, high in fiber and low in fat. The diet incorporating the American Cancer Society guidelines is discussed in Chapter 6. There is also information on antioxidants and the best sources of vitamins A, C and E in Chapter 9.

Menus

1,500 Calorie

Breakfast
1 banana bran muffin
1 cup 1% milk
1 orange

Lunch
Hummus plus 4 pita chips
Tossed salad with 1 cup lettuce
1/2 cup grated carrots and vinegar
1 white bread dinner roll
1 cup watermelon

Dinner
3 grilled portabello mushrooms
4 oz grilled salmon
Tossed salad with 1 cup lettuce,
    1/2 cup grated carrots, vinegar
1 white dinner roll
1 cup watermelon

2,000 Calorie

Breakfast
2 eggs scrambled burrito w/ onions, spinach, bell peppers
1 cup orange juice
2 slices wheat toast
1/2 banana

Lunch
1 cup spinach & potato cream soup
Caesar salad with croutons: 1 cup Romaine lettuce; 1/3 cup low fat grated parmesan; 1 tsp. olive oil
Chicken sandwich on 2 slices of whole wheat bread
1 cup skim milk
1 bunch of grapes
1/2 cup frozen yogurt

Dinner
1 cup black bean soup
1 white dinner roll
oven roasted vegetables:
   1 bell pepper, sweet potatoes, 1 onion, garlic

chicken cacciatore
1 cup sherbet

iv. Diet for Diabetics

Diabetes—"preventing this potential killer does not call for a sugar free diet" (Sharp, 1998), but some discretions are necessary. A good diabetic diet should have the following nutritional goals (ADA, 1999):

1. Maintain near normal blood glucose
2. Achieve normal lipid levels
3. Provide adequate calories
4. Prevent low sugar levels
5. Improve overall health

    Let us look at some basic information about carbohydrates and diabetic diet. Fifty-five to sixty percent of the daily calorie intake should come from carbohydrates, ten to twenty percent from protein, less than ten percent from saturated fat, less than ten percent from polyunsaturated fats and sixty to seventy percent from monounsaturated fats and carbohydrates. Most carbohydrates are converted to glucose within two hours after eating. Avoid items rich in sugars such as soft drinks, fruit juices, and desserts. They overload your pancreas. One gram of carbohydrates gives four calories. Foods with carbohydrates include:

> Fruits and vegetables
> Grain products—bread, pasta, rice, oats, cereals, cookies, crackers
> Beans, peas, lentils
> Dairy products—milk and yogurt
> Sugar and sugar-sweetened foods

If you are an insulin-dependent diabetic, eat at consistent times synchronized with insulin injection, and monitor blood glucose levels carefully. Adjust insulin doses for the amount of food eaten. Consult a diabetes care provider for precise advice or medication.

If you are a diabetic not on insulin, eat a low fat diet of 250–500 fewer calories than the average daily intake and increase your physical activity. Space your meals to spread carbohydrate intake throughout the day.

If you fall in the categories of requiring 1,500 calories or 2,000 calories daily, the following menus will help. But remember that carbohydrate snacks are important in preventing hypoglycemia especially if you are on diabetes medications.

Menus

1,500 Calories

Breakfast
1 bagel with 1 1/2 Tbl
　low fat cream cheese
1 cup strawberries
1 cup 1% milk

Dinner
2 oz sirloin steak
1/2 baked potato
1 tsp. margarine

Lunch
1 cup tomato soup
3 slices of turkey
2 slices of wheat bread
1 leaf of lettuce

1/2 cup boiled corn
1 cup 1% milk
1 frozen fruit juice bar

2,000 Calories

Breakfast
1 inch slice of banana bread
1 tsp. margarine
1 cup low fat yogurt
1 orange
1 cup fat free milk

Lunch
6 oz grilled chicken
Tossed salad: 1 cup lettuce,
1 cup tomato
1 Tbl. reduced fat dressing
1/2 cup watermelon
6 oz orange juice

Dinner
6 oz baked chicken
1 wheat bread roll
1 cup roasted vegetables
1 cup mixed fruit
6 oz fruit juice

v. Hypoglycemia Diet

Over 20 million Americans suffer from hypoglycemia. The normal blood sugar level is 65mg/dl to 115mg/dl. If blood sugar levels should drop below 50mg/dl, you develop the condition called hypoglycemia, and you experience the symptoms of sweating, dizziness, palpitations, tremors, hunger, fatigue, headache, restlessness, nervousness, light-headedness, blurred vision, anxiety and fainting.

The general objective in the treatment of hypoglycemia is to control the elevation of blood sugars which cause subsequent excessive hypoglycemic rebounds for reactive or spontaneous hypoglycemia. Diet therapy is effective and is the mainstay of treatment. For a person suffering from hypoglycemia the diet should be high in protein and low in carbohydrates, with 120–140 g of protein, 75–100 g of carbohydrates and sufficient fat to maintain ideal body weight. The food intake should be distributed in six small meals per day. Therefore, wolfing down a big meal or skipping other meals would be a big mistake. This would throw the sugar levels out of whack and worsen hypoglycemia. It is important to select the right food items to create six meals. Eat regularly, select a variety of foods and limit the intake of caffeine.

Use the following items in generous amounts:

a) Poached, Scrambled, soft or hard boiled eggs
b) Cheese of any kind (except whey cheese)
c) Vegetables, such as asparagus, sprouts, broccoli, cabbage, cauliflower, celery, cucumbers, radishes and tomatoes
d) Broth type soups containing vegetables and lean meats
e) Plain gelatin desserts
f) Artificially sweetened jelly
g) Butter, margarine, mayonnaise
h) Artificially sweetened carbonated drinks.

The following items are permitted but in limited amounts:

a) Milk, buttermilk, plain yogurt
b) Cottage cheese
c) Artichokes, beets, carrots
d) Fresh fruits or unsweetened fruits
e) Bread (1 slice), bagel (1/2), muffin and graham crackers
f) Artificially sweetened pudding or custard
g) Fruit juices without added sugar or substitutes for fruits.

But avoid the following items:

a) Vegetable protein meat substitutes
b) Corn, potatoes, sweet potatoes
c) Fruits canned in sugar syrup
d) Pancakes, waffles, sweet rolls, coffee cakes and donuts
e) Sweetened gelatin, custards and puddings
f) Jelly, sugar, honey and candy
g) Alcohol
h) Regularly sweetened carbonated drinks.

Menus

1500 Calories

Breakfast
2 eggs
1 slice of bread
1 tsp. margarine
carbonated drink

Mid-Morning Snack
1 cup skim milk

Lunch
3 ounces lean meat or tuna
1/2 stalk of celery or 1 tomato
3 cheese crackers
1 tsp. margarine
1 orange

Mid-Afternoon Snack
1 cup yogurt

Dinner
1 cup fresh spinach
3 oz broiled chicken, pork or beef
1/2 cup cooked peas
1 slice garlic bread w/ 1 tsp. butter or margarine
1/2 cup plain gelatin

Bedtime Snack
1 cup skim milk

2000 Calories

Breakfast
2 eggs
2 slices of bacon
1 slice of bread or 1/2 cup cereal
carbonated drink

Mid-Morning Snack
1 small hot dog or sausage

Lunch
4 ounces lean meat or tuna
1 cup broccoli or asparagus
1/2 cup cucumbers
  or cooked cabbage
6 crackers
2 tsp. margarine
1 cup grapes

Mid-Afternoon Snack
2 ounces of peanuts

Dinner
1 cup spinach salad
1 Tbl. Italian dressing
4 oz of fish, chicken or turkey
1 oz cheddar cheese
1/2 cup cooked peas or beans
   w/ 1 tsp. margarine
1/2 cup plain gelatin

Bedtime Snack
1 cup skim milk
2 crackers

vi. Anti-Gout Diet

High uric acid (purine) can lead to gout. These levels are generally controlled by medication, but can be helped by following an appropriate diet.

1. Avoid high fat meats and desserts.
2. Eat less beef, lamb, pork, eggs and regular cheese.
3. Prefer fish and poultry.
4. Avoid deep fried foods.

Some foods are high in purine. Avoid them. These foods include:

Anchovies	Organs (e.g. liver, heart, kidney)
Herring	Mackerel
Sardines	Scallops
Sweetbreads	Goose
Alcoholic beverages	Meat broth, drippings or gravy

Choose from the following items which are very low in purine:

non-fat buttermilk	cottage cheese
coffee/ tea	breads
cocoa	salt
carbonated drinks	fruits and fruit juices
candies/sugar/honey	sherbet

Menus

1,500 Calories

Breakfast
1/2 banana
1 cup cornflakes
1 slice wheat toast
1 tsp. margarine
6 oz orange juice

Lunch
6 oz tomato soup
1 orange
2 oz cheddar cheese
2 slices white bread
1 cup 1% milk

Dinner
3 oz halibut with parsley and lemon
1/2 cup steamed rice
1/2 cup broccoli
1 dinner roll
3 oz orange sherbet

2,000 Calories

Breakfast
1 cup strawberries
1 cup low fat yogurt
1 cup 1% milk
1 scrambled egg
1 slice white toast

Lunch
6 oz tomato soup
1 cup salad with 1/2 tomato
1 Tbl. Italian dressing
4 crackers/saltines
1 oz cheddar cheese
1 cup watermelon
6 oz fruit juice

Dinner
4 oz grilled chicken
1 corn on the cob
1 tsp. margarine
1/2 cup rice
3 spears of asparagus
1 cup fruit salad
1 frozen yogurt bar

vii. Low Salt Diet

A low salt diet is used for people who have high blood pressure, have a family history of hypertension or who are suffering from heart failure and fluid retention. To get the correct amount of salt in your diet it is critical to learn:

1. What labels mean
2. Which foods are high in sodium
3. Which seasonings and sauces are loaded with sodium
4. What are the ways to enhance flavor without adding salt

Be aware that sodium-free means less than a 5 mg sodium per serving, very low sodium means less than 35 mg per serving, low sodium means less than 140 mg and unsalted means no salt added.

The following foods are high in sodium:

bacon	buttermilk	dry cereal
cheese	potato chips	crackers
frankfurters/sausages	cured meats	corned meats
processed meats	salted nuts/ seeds	green olives
pickles	pizza	sauerkraut
canned soups		

The seasonings and sauces with a lot of salt include:

soy sauce	chili sauce	worcestershire sauce
meat tenderizer	steak sauce	bouillon cubes
ketchup	seasoning salts	

Look for low salt versions of these items. (Table 8.1 gives the amounts of sodium in common drinks.) If you want to enhance the flavor of the food without using salt try these ideas (Starke and Winston, 1990):

1. Toast seeds and nuts to bring out flavor.
2. Roast vegetables.
3. Grate and use fruit skins.

TABLE 8.1
The Nutritional Value of Ten Common Drinks

Item	Amount	Calories	Vit A I.U.	Vit C mg	Sodium mg
Spring Water	1 liter	0	N/A	N/A	2-20
Whole Milk	1 cup	150	350	3.3	120
2% Milk	1 cup	120	500	2.8	122
Skim milk	1 cup	86	500	2.5	126
Iced Tea w/ lemon & sugar	1 cup	70	N/A	N/A	0
Coffee	6 oz	4	N/A	N/A	0-2
Coke	6 oz	72	N/A	N/A	7
Pepsi	6 oz	80	N/A	N/A	2
Orange Juice	1 cup	80	N/A	72	N/A
Grapefruit Juice	6 oz	80	N/A	60	10
Tomato Juice	6 oz	30	N/A	25	500
Apple juice	6 oz	90	N/A	100	N/A

4. Use fresh herbs instead of dried.
5. Sprinkle vinegar or citrus juice.
6. Use dry or salt-free mustard.
7. Add fresh hot peppers.
8. Use herbs and spices to season vegetables.
9. Use freshly ground spices.

Menus

1,500 Calorie

Breakfast
1 cup sliced bananas
1 cup skim milk
1/2 cup plain low fat yogurt
1 egg
1 tsp. unsalted margarine

Dinner
4 oz broiled salmon
1 tsp. margarine
6 spears of asparagus

Lunch
Chicken with rice
small tossed salad: 1 cup lettuce &
    1 slice tomato
1/2 cup frozen yogurt
1 orange

1 whole wheat dinner role
1 1/2 cups watermelon
1 cup fresh strawberries

2,000 Calorie

Breakfast
3 pancakes with maple syrup
1 cup orange juice
1/2 cup 1% milk
1/2 banana

Dinner
3 oz sirloin steak
4 fresh mushrooms
1/2 cup steamed green beans
1 cup orange sherbet

Lunch
Spaghetti w/ mushroom sauce
1 white bread roll
1 cup steamed broccoli
1/2 piece angel food cake

1 tossed salad with 1 cup
    lettuce & 1 slice tomato
1 cup skim milk

viii. High Fiber Diet

Fiber simply speeds the passage of food through the digestive tract and dilutes carcinogens. This is the way it prevents constipation and reduces the risk of diverticulosis, and colon cancer. The soluble fiber also helps lower cholesterol. A good intake of fiber is about 20 – 25 grams daily of which 25% should be soluble and 75% insoluble. You can get soluble fiber from oats, beans and barley and the insoluble fiber is in abundance in whole grain bread, brown rice, bran cereal, fruits and vegetables (Sheasby, 1997). Refer to Table 8.2 for the amounts of fiber in ten best sources.

Menus

1,500 Calories

Breakfast
2 slices banana bran loaf
1 cup 1% milk
1 grapefruit

Lunch
Tossed salad with 1 cup lettuce
1/2 cup grated carrots
2 tsp. low calorie french dressing
1 wheat roll
dried fruit

Dinner
4 oz salmon
2 oz broccoli pilaf
fresh tomato and lentil soup

Caesar salad with croutons
6 oz fruit juice
1 slice pineapple upside down cake

2,000 Calories

Breakfast
1 Raisin Bran muffin
6 oz orange juice
1/2 cup low fat yogurt
    with nectarine slices

Lunch
1 baked potato w/ 2 tsp margarine
1 oz cheddar cheese
6 oz chicken and bean casserole
1 cup fruit salad
1 cup 1% milk

Dinner
6 oz chicken or fish
fresh cooked green beans, peas
1 cup low fat yogurt
    with fresh strawberries

1 wheat roll
beans and brown rice

TABLE 8.2

Ten Best Sources of Fiber

Item	Amount of Fiber in a 100 g Serving
Bran Bread	8.6 g
Bran cereal	35.2
Bran flakes	18.8
Oatmeal	10.6
Barley (raw)	15.6
Whole Grain Cornbread	11.0
Wheat Bran	15.0
Baked Beans	7.7
Almonds	11.2
Pistachios	10.8

ix. High Calcium Diet

Your bones are the depository of calcium, and like a bank, they gain and lose reserves constantly, to maintain the right levels of calcium. Requirements of calcium at different ages are presented in Chapter 9. A good reference work on calcium is *The Calcium Cookbook* (Ness and Subak-Sharpe, 1998). A few simple facts are worth remembering:

1. Excess of bran, salt and caffeine may interfere with calcium absorption
2. Don't use vegetables only for a calcium supply, since calcium from these is not always absorbed well
3. Take calcium supplements if you have lactose intolerance or are allergic to dairy products.

Menus

1,500 Calories

Breakfast
6 oz orange juice
1 cup low fat yogurt
1/2 cup cereal
1 cup 1% milk
1/2 banana

Dinner
4 stuffed mushrooms
Baked fish and potato
1 dinner roll

Lunch
Salmon quiche
1 cup spinach salad with
   1/2 cup chick peas
1 slice white bread
1 orange

1 piece streusel coffee cake
6 oz fruit juice

2,000 Calories

Breakfast
2 buttermilk pancakes
1 English muffin/ 1 tsp. margarine
1 banana
1/2 cup low fat yogurt
1 cup 1% milk

Dinner
2 cheese enchiladas
1/2 cup watermelon
1 cup yogurt & fruit parfait

Lunch
Cream of vegetable soup
1 wheat bread roll
Spaghetti with cheese sauce
1 cup yogurt and fruit parfait
6 oz of orange juice

Lentil soup
6 oz fruit juice
1 cup salad w/ sliced tomato

x. Bland (Ulcer) Diet

Bland diets are recommended for patients who have irritation of the lining of the stomach from an ulcer or gastritis. A high gastric acid secretion is a major factor in causing stomach and duodenal ulcers. To prevent or reduce acid secretion try to avoid the following items:

1. Cheese with added spices, nuts, relishes
2. Salted or smoked lunch meats and frankfurters
3. Fried meat, chicken or fish
4. Raw vegetable, e.g. cabbage, broccoli, garlic, beans
5. Highly seasoned creamed soups and broth
6. Fruits with skins, raisins, pineapple
7. Whole grain cereals, bread, crackers
8. Pies, pastries, candies, chocolates
9. Spicy, seasoned dressings, sauces, curries, spices
10. Coffee, tea, alcoholic and carbonated beverages

Remember these tips: Eat slowly and chew thoroughly. Eat meals at the same hour each day. Eat protein rich foods. Sip citrus juices during meals so they are well mixed with food. Eating snacks during mornings or afternoons helps in preventing increased acid secretion. The amount of snacking should be based on desired caloric intake e.g. graham crackers with peanut butter, pudding and saltines.

References

American Diabetic Association (1999). Nutrition recommendations and principles for people with diabetes mellitus: American Diabetic Association position statement. *Diabetes Care, vol 22*, suppl: 42-5.

American Heart Association (1996). Dietary guidelines for healthy American adults. Website: http://www.amhrt.org.

Baily, C. and Bishop, L. (1995). *Fit or Fat Target Recipes*. Boston, MA: Houghton Mifflin.

Ness, J. and Subak-Sharpe, G. (1998). *The Calcium Cookbook*. NY, NY: M. Evans & Co.

Sharp, D. (1998, April). Can a customized diet reduce inherited risk. *Hippocrates, 53*.

Sheasby, A. (1997). *My Fiber Cookbook*. New York, NY: Anness Publishing, Ltd.

Starke, R.D. and Winston, M. (1990). *American Heart Association Low Salt Cookbook, A Complete Guide to Reducing Sodium and Fat in the Diet*. New York, NY: Times Books, Division of Random House, Inc.

Section III.
Magic Bullets

Chapter 9

❧ ❧

Who Says There Are No Magic Bullets? Eight Of Them Are Right Here

In 1997, thirty-five percent of Americans believed vitamin supplements were necessary, and, in that year, they spent $ 5.7 billion on supplements—an amount that has more than doubled since 1990 (Center for Science in the Public Interest, 1998). Seventy percent of Americans use supplements at least occasionally (Newsweek, 1993). High impact advertising and conflicting information have created significant confusion in the minds of the population; many are not able to separate good scientific information from hype and hysteria.

Antioxidants: The Three Aces

Antioxidants protect the body cells and tissues from assaults by free radicals. Free radicals are molecules which lack an essential component called an electron. They become harmful when they steal an electron from another molecule causing damage to cells. Damage from free radicals contributes to disorders like heart disease, stroke, cancer and cataracts and also to the aging process. The free radicals are produced during normal physiological functions, from trauma, inflammation, drugs and radiation.

Vitamins C, E, and beta carotene (a precursor of vitamin A) are antioxidant vitamins. Vitamins are substances other than proteins, carbohydrates, fats, minerals and salts, which are essential for the normal metabolism, growth and development of the body. Currently a common strategy for longevity is the use of antioxidants. There is no doubt that vitamin C, E and beta carotene are good antioxidants, but should we get them from foods or supplements? The answer follows the analysis of the latest studies.

i. Vitamin A

Vitamin A is an important antioxidant and immune system enhancer. It is present in fish and meats. We can also get it from vegetables in the precursor form, beta carotene. The liver and intestines convert beta carotene to vitamin A.

Ten functions of Vitamin A

1. As an antioxidant it controls free radicals and functions as an anti-cancer agent.
2. It enhances the immune system by maintaining a healthy thymus gland.
3. It participates in synthesis of RNA.
4. It maintains health of new skin and the mucous membranes.
5. It promotes night vision, prevents blindness.
6. It maintains metabolism of tissue.
7. It participates in reproduction and lactation cycles.
8. It helps in the prevention of inflammatory prostaglandin release.
9. It takes part in prevention of degenerative diseases.
10. It promotes growth of healthy bones and teeth.

Deficiency and Overdose

The consequences of vitamin A deficiency are reflected in a table in the appendix (Appendix B, Table 1). Night blindness is the earliest symptom of deficiency.

TABLE 9.1

Ten Best Sources of Vitamin A

Daily Requirement:	For Men: 1000 mcg RE For Women: 800 mcg RE
Item	Serving
Liver (beef, pork)	12 oz
Liver (chicken)	2 oz
Oatmeal	10 cups
Cereal	4 oz
Apricots	2 cups
Cantaloupe	2 oz
Mangoes	2 cups
Broccoli, Spinach	2 cups
Carrots, Peas, Peppers	2 cups
Skim Milk	8 cups

How much do you need?

For men 1000 mcg and for women 800 mcg daily. The signs and symptoms of overdosing are presented in Appendix B, Table 1.

Should you take supplements?

The current research data do not support the use of supplements. You will find more information in the discussion of latest studies presented below. Table 9.1 gives you the ten best sources. It lists the items and serving sizes that will give you the recommended daily allowance (RDA).

TABLE 9.2

Ten Best Sources of Vitamin C

Daily Requirement:	For Men: 60 mg RE For Women: 60 mg RE
Item	Serving
Liver (beef, pork)	12 oz
Cereal	4 oz
Sweet Potatoes	4 medium size
Asparagus, Broccoli, Peppers	2 cups
Cantaloupe	2 oz
Grapefruit	2 cups
Mangoes	2 medium size
Orange	4 medium size
Strawberries	2 cups
Grapes, Oranges	3 cups

ii. Vitamin C

Vitamin C is a powerful antioxidant that affects almost all the body functions. It is important because of its many versatile actions.

Ten functions of Vitamin C

1. It detoxifies harmful free radical substances.
2. It strengthens the immune system.
3. It promotes wound healing.
4. It plays a key role in the promotion of strong bones and teeth.
5. It has a role in the synthesis of proteins.
6. It helps metabolize calcium and folic acid and aids iron absorption.
7. It helps lower the levels of cholesterol and uric acid.

8. It functions as an antagonistic agent and helps fight infections.
9. It helps promote recovery from heart attacks.
10. It is essential for the development and maintenance of connective tissue. It fights aging and extends life.

Deficiency and Overdose

The signs and symptoms of deficiency and overdose are summarized in Appendix B, Table 1.

How much should you take?

The current RDA for vitamin C is 60 mg daily for men and women. This figure was set in 1989. This RDA is now under revision by the Food and Nutrition Board of the National Academy of Sciences. The experts are recommending that the RDA be raised to 100–200 mg per day. This amount is safe and will prevent deficiency symptoms and signs. Table 9.2 gives you the ten best sources of vitamin C. It lists the items and the serving sizes that will give you the RDA of 60 mg. However, to get 100-200 mg of vitamin C take five servings of fruits and vegetables daily (Levine, 1999). Such intake is considered beneficial in preventing cancer.

iii. Vitamin E

This is another powerful antioxidant that protects your body, cell membranes, and the genetic material in cells. It protects ingested nutrients from oxidation and free radical attacks. With these functions Vitamin E is used in cases of hardening of the arteries, thrombophlebitis, abnormal blood clotting, cystic breast disease, and the bends suffered by divers.

Ten functions of Vitamin E

1. It is a free radical fighting antioxidant, and has a role in promoting a balance in prostaglandins.
2. It is a potent antioxidant against LDL oxidation; retards arterial plaque and reduces artery blockage.
3. It rejuvenates the immune system.

4. It protects DNA from free radical oxidation.
5. It protects fatty acids from breaking down.
6. It protects the coverings (myelin nerve sheaths) of nerves.
7. It maintains vitamin C and vitamin B from oxidation.
8. It relieves arthritic pain.
9. It protects the pituitary and adrenal hormones.
10. It strengthens heart muscle.

Deficiency and Overdose

The signs and symptoms of vitamin E deficiency and overdose are summarized in Table 1 in Appendix B.

Ten Best Sources of Vitamin E

Table 9.3 lists the sources and the serving sizes that will provide you with the Recommended Daily Allowance of vitamin E.

Foods That Do It All

Finally, here is a list of ten items that are the best sources of all three antioxidants-vitamins A, C, and E: Tomatoes, garlic, soy, grapes, broccoli, cranberries, cayenne, green tea, licorice, and blueberries.

Latest Studies: Positive and Negative Results

Beta Carotene and Vitamin A—Supplements Not Beneficial. A study of 18,314 smokers, former smokers and workers exposed to asbestos who were given 30 mg of beta carotene and 25,000 IU of Vitamin A led to this conclusion: "After an average of four years of supplementation, the combination of beta carotene and vitamin A had no benefit and may have had adverse effect on the incidence of lung cancer and on the risk of death from lung cancer, cardiovascular disease, and any cause in smokers and workers exposed to asbestos" (New England Journal of Medicine, 1996).

Vitamins A, C and E—Supplements Not Beneficial to Post-Menopausal Women: A study of 34,486 postmenopausal women indicated "there was little evidence that the intake of vitamin E from supplements was associated with a decreased risk of death from coronary artery disease...

TABLE 9.3
Ten Best Sources of Vitamin E

Daily Requirement:	For Men:10 mcg RE For Women:8 mcg RE
Item	Serving
Shrimp	12 oz
Cereal	4 oz
Plain Wheat Germ	8 Tbl
Apricots, Peaches	4 cups
Greens	4 cups
Almonds	8 Tbl
Peanut Butter	8 Tbl
Sunflower Seeds	8 Tbl
Sweet Potatoes	4 medium size
Mayonnaise	1 Tbl

the intake of vitamin A and C was not associated with lower risks of dying from coronary disease." Advice from this study: Postmenopausal women can lower their risk of coronary artery disease without using vitamin supplements (Kushi et al, 1996).

Vitamins A, C, and E—Supplements Do Not Prevent Colorectal Cancer: In a four year clinical trial of 751 patients, vitamin C (1 g) and beta carotene (25 mg) or beta carotene plus vitamin C and E were given. There was no evidence of either beta carotene or vitamins C and E causing reduction in the incidence of colorectal adenoma. The conclusion was that the lack of efficacy of these vitamins argues against the use of supplemental vitamin C and E and beta carotene to prevent colorectal cancer (Greenberg, 1994).

Vitamins A and E—Supplements Do Not Reduce Lung Cancer. There was no reduction in the incidence of lung cancer among 29,133 male smokers, age 50–59, who were given 50 mg of alpha-tocopherol (vitamin E) and 20 mg of beta carotene (vitamin A) per day for a period of 5–8 years (New England Journal of Medicine, 1994).

Vitamins C or E—Large Doses Do Not Prevent Breast Cancer. A study of 89,494 women age 34–59 showed that large dosages of vitamin C or E did not protect participants from breast cancer (Hunter et al, 1993).

Vitamin A—Supplements Not Beneficial to Prevent Cancer or Heart Disease: A study of 22,071 physicians age 40–84 who were given 50 mg of beta carotene on alternate days for 12 years concluded that the supplementation "produced neither benefit nor harm in terms of the incidence of malignant neoplasms (cancer), cardiovascular disease or death from all causes" (New England Journal of Medicine, 1996).

Vitamin E—Supplements Reduce Risk of Heart Attacks. The Cambridge Heart Antioxidant Study (CHAOS) studied 2002 men and women with atherosclerosis. They were given vitamin E supplements (400 IU or 800 IU) or placebo daily. After 17 months of using the supplements, the risk of non-fatal heart attacks was reduced by 77%. The risk of fatal heart attacks was also significantly reduced (Cambridge Heart Antioxidant Study, 1996).

Vitamins A and E—Supplements Do Not Prevent Coronary Heart Disease: A study of 27,271 male smokers age 50–69 with no history of heart attacks were given 50 mcg of vitamin E and 20 mg of beta carotene daily for 5–8 years. The result: no conclusive evidence that supplemental vitamin E reduces the risk of coronary artery disease and it is unlikely that beta carotene has a notable role in the prevention of coronary artery disease. Conclusion: There are no grounds to recommend supplemental vitamin E or beta carotene to prevent coronary artery disease (Virtamo et al, 1998).

Vitamins A or E—Supplements Do Not Decrease Heart Attacks. A study of 1,862 male smokers age 50–69 indicated that the number of major coronary events, in men with previous heart attacks, did not decrease with the supplements of vitamin E or beta carotene (Rapola et al, 1997).

Vitamin A—Bad for Lung Cancer; Vitamin E—Good for Prostate Cancer: A recent review of medical records of thousands of smokers indicated a reduced risk of prostate cancer by a third with the use of Vitamin E. The uses of beta carotene in this study showed that they were 16% more likely to develop cancer. Advice from the study: It is premature to recommend that everybody start taking vitamin E supplements (Sun Sentinel, 3/18/98).

Vitamins A, C and E—Do Not Help the Heart An editorial in the New England Journal of Medicine states that recent studies have found "inverse association between the frequency of coronary artery disease and dietary intake of antioxidant vitamins." (Diaz et al, 1997).

What Does All This Mean?

Conclusions on the basis of hard facts:

1. Vitamin E supplements may lower the incidence of prostate cancer.
2. Vitamin A (beta carotene) supplements may increase the risk of lung cancer.
3. Persons over the age of 80 have been found to have lower levels of antioxidants.
4. Beta carotene taken as a single nutrient in large amounts may produce adverse effects.
5. Grains and beans are excellent sources of many vitamins and minerals.
6. You can get all the vitamins and minerals you need by eating a whole variety of foods. Foods contain the ideal mix of nutrients.
7. Nutrient imbalances and toxicities are less likely to occur when nutrients are derived from foods.
8. Most nutrient toxicities occur through supplementation. Table 1, Appendix B indicates signs and symptoms of deficiency and overdose.

9. The available evidence supports the use of Vitamin E supplements in persons with risk factors for heart disease. But the risk of stroke may increase in patients with high blood pressure (Wolf and Wolf, 1998).

Should You Take Vitamin and Mineral Supplements?

The current evidence for taking supplemental antioxidants is not convincing. The conclusions of professionals with the responsible large national organizations is that further studies should be done before concrete recommendations can be made for the supplemental use of antioxidants.

The American Medical Association and the American Cancer Society offer no specific recommendations except to follow the advice to get recommended daily allowances (RDA) of these vitamins. The advice of the American Dietetic Association is the most prudent and sensible:

1. It is best to get all nutrients from foods.
2. Use supplementation of B-12 for strict vegetarians who eliminate all animal products from diet.
3. Use supplementation of folic acid for women of child bearing age who consume limited amounts of fruits, vegetables, and legumes.
4. Use supplementation of vitamin D for persons with limited milk intake and sunlight exposure.
5. Use supplementation of calcium for persons with lactose intolerance or allergies to dairy products.
6. Use supplementation of multivitamins and minerals for persons following severely restricted weight-loss diets. Use multivitamin supplements if you are on a weight loss program using Xenical.
7. Use beta carotene 50 mg on alternate days if you are over 65 years of age.
8. Take Thiamine 50 mg daily if your alcohol consumption is more than moderate.
9. If you are a smoker take supplements of Vitamin C 500 mg, vitamin E 100 IU and beta carotene 20 mg daily
10. Remember the new RDA for vitamin C is 100-200 mg.

Supplements should be used only if there is clear proof of benefits. Supplements of antioxidants in large doses should be used only if they are proven not to be toxic. Until this is accomplished, stay off popping those pills and follow the guaranteed preventive measures of cholesterol-lowering diet, regular exercise and smoking cessation.

iv. Vitamin D: The Sunshine Vitamin

1. Vitamin D is important for bone development in children and bone maintenance in adults. It is essential for preventing osteoporosis and bone fractures in elderly.
2. The sun is a big source. Vitamin D is also found in egg yolks, fatty fish, fish oils and fortified margarine and milk.
3. The Food and Nutrition Board, The Institute of Medicine and The National Academy of Science recently issued new guidelines and they recommended daily allowance of vitamin D (RDA) for adults as follows: 19–50 years, 200 IU; 51–10 years, 400 IU; over 71 years, 600 IU.
4. Don't be over enthusiastic in taking vitamin D. It can be dangerous. Make sure you don't go over the recommended limits. Toxic effects can occur when daily doses exceed 1,000 IU with symptoms of muscle weakness, headache, nausea, vomiting, malaise, lethargy, abdominal pain and constipation. The doses in the range of 2,000 IU can cause irreversible damage to the kidneys and heart. For signs and symptoms of deficiency and overdose, see Appendix B, Table 1.
5. The factors that increase vitamin D deficiency are: inadequate sun exposure, poor diet, chronic liver disease, chronic kidney disease and treatment with anti-coagulants.
6. It is possible to be deficient and not know it. Thirty to forty percent of adults over the age of 50 are either borderline or overtly vitamin D deficient and have no symptoms of deficiency (Center for Science in the Public Interest, 1998).
7. In children the inability to absorb Vitamin D can cause rickets, a combination of weak muscles, delayed tooth development and

weaker, softer bones. In adults, the deficiency can cause osteomalacia, a condition in which the bones are softer, more porous and liable to fracture easily.
8. Deficiency may remain symptomless for decades and may be detected after a lot of damage is done to bones. Too late to catch up? One study of elderly subjects concluded that the persons who took 700 IU of vitamin D and 500 mg of calcium daily were less than half as likely as control subjects to sustain a fracture (Dawson-Hughes, et al, 1997).
9. Vitamin D is more than a cousin of calcium. It is like a twin. You need vitamin D to help absorb calcium in food. When persons do not get enough vitamin D in their diet they are not able to absorb dietary calcium efficiently. Thus, vitamin D and calcium go hand-in-hand to strengthen your bones and teeth.
10. Age makes a big difference in vitamin D absorption. Older people are less sun exposed. Also, aging makes the skin less efficient in converting ultraviolet light to vitamin D. This is why older folks are more at risk for vitamin D deficiency and require higher amounts of vitamin D obtainable from skim milk or cheese.

v. Don't be a Jellyfish, Bone Up on Calcium

Catch on about calcium. Here are ten important facts to remember:

1. Calcium is the most abundant mineral in the body. It is found mostly in your bones, and there is some in the blood.
2. The body does not produce calcium: you must get it from diet.
3. Calcium gives strength to bones, helps muscles contract and your heart beat and it regulates nerve function.
4. Calcium depleted bones become porous and fragile and fracture easily. This is osteoporosis. It affects one in four women and one in eight men over the age of 50.
5. Osteoporosis is preventable. Regular physical activity and a diet adequate in calcium are the best preventive measures.
6. Calcium needs are highest during childhood and adolescence for bone growth.

TABLE 9.4

Ten Best Sources of Calcium

Daily Requirement:	For Men: 800-1200 mcg RE For Women: 800-1200 mcg RE
Item	Serving
Milk	8 oz
Yogurt	8 oz
Bran, English Muffin	4 oz
Broccoli, Spinach	8 oz
Swiss Cheese	1 oz
Cheddar Cheese	1.5 oz
Monterey Cheese	2 oz
Ricotta Cheese	4 oz
Ice Cream	8 oz
Tofu	4 oz

7. Pregnant and breast feeding women and postmenopausal women have high calcium needs to minimize bone loss.
8. Three out of four adult women do not meet the current recommended daily intake for calcium.
9. Vitamin D helps absorb the calcium in food and deposit it in bones and teeth. So you must get enough vitamin D from the sun and fortified food.
10. Close the calcium gap. Get it from sources shown in Table 9.4. Other good sources are: seafood (3 oz contain 181 mg), buttermilk (1 cup contains 285 mg), figs (5 contain 135 mg), and almonds (80 mg in 1 oz). Get enough to meet the new calcium recommendations listed in Table 9.5.

TABLE 9.5

Calcium: Recommended Daily Requirement

Age (year)	RDA
Birth - 6 mo	400 mg
6 mo - 1 yr	600 mg
1 - 5 yr	800 mg
6 - 10 yr	800 - 1200 mg
11 - 24 yr	1200 - 1500 mg
Pregnant Adolescents	2000 mg
Pregnant Women	1200 - 1500 mg
Women 25 - menopause	800 - 1200 mg
Post-menopausal Women on Estrogen	1000 mg
Post-menopausal Women not on Estrogen	800 - 1200 mg
Men 25 - 65	800 - 1200 mg
Men 65 +	1500 mg

vi. Folate: For The Jolly Green Giant

The name folic acid comes from the Latin word folium meaning leaf. Folic acid is an essential B vitamin. It has several functions:

1. Basic maintenance of blood and immune system
2. Synthesis of DNA and RNA
3. Production and maturation of red and white blood cells
4. Prevention and treatment of some anemias
5. Metabolism of proteins and synthesis of amino acids.

How does folate help humans? Recent literature claims that folic acid can enhance brain function, prevent heart attacks, alleviate anemia, ward off mental degeneration, retard aging, help prevent and cure depression, help block and reverse cancer, and help prevent birth defects such as spina bifida.

Deficiency of folic acid can cause megaloblastic anemia. Deficiency can be caused by poor dietary intake of fresh fruits and vegetables, impaired absorption as a result of damage to the proximal small intestine from a condition called sprue, and increased loss caused by hemodialysis. Nursing mothers, pregnant women and individuals with hyperthyroidism or alcoholism require an increased intake of folic acid.

The best sources of folates are green vegetables, the richest being asparagus, broccoli, spinach and lettuce. Each contains more than 1 mg of folate per 100 g of dry weight. See Table 9.6 for ten best sources. Other sources are liver, kidney, yeast and mushrooms. It should be noted that cooking destroys a lot of folic acid. The RDA ranges from 25–400 mcg, depending on age, sex, and other factors.

How much is too much?

Up to 400 mcg of folic acid can be obtained from your diet. Intakes of over 5,000 mcg of folic acid per day could mask symptoms of B12 deficiency and pernicious anemia. For recommended daily requirements, see Table 9.7.

Elevated levels of a blood protein, homocysteine, are considered to be a factor for heart disease. Folic acid can help free enzymes to metabolize homocysteine and this decreases the chances of heart disease. A study of 80,082 women from 1980 to 1994 lead to this conclusion: "The intake of folate and vitamin B6 above the current recommended dietary allowance may be important in the primary prevention of coronary artery disease in women" (JAMA, 1998).

vii. Zinc: A Miracle Mineral

Zinc represents only 0.003% of the human body, amounting to 1.4-2.3 g. It is an intrinsic part of at least 110 metalloenzymes and other cellular components (Wyngarden and Smith, 1988). Zinc is an essential mineral

TABLE 9.6

Ten Best Sources of Folate

Daily Requirement:	For Men: 180 mcg RE For Women: 200 mcg RE
Item	Serving
Beef Liver	12 oz
Whole Wheat Muffin	8 oz
Cereal	4 oz
Greens	4 cups
Beans, Peas, Lentils	2 cups
Asparagus, Beets	4 cups
Broccoli, Brussels Sprouts	4 cups
Cauliflower	4 cups
Cabbage, Corn	4 cups
Spinach	4 cups

for the synthesis of protein, DNA and RNA. Ninety-nine percent of zinc is inside cells. The highest concentrations are in the prostate, skin and its appendages, brain, choroid, liver, pancreas, bone, and blood.

Where do we get zinc?

Good sources are unrefined grains, bran flakes, rice, corn, peas, potatoes, spinach, oatmeal, and legumes. Sources of zinc and other minerals are identified in Table 9.8 and 9.9. Zinc requirements of a developing fetus, pregnant woman and growing child or adolescent are higher than that of an adult man or non-pregnant woman.

Zinc is absorbed from the small intestine and excreted mainly in the feces and a small amount in the urine. Zinc deficiency may occur

TABLE 9.7
Folates: Recommended Daily Requirement

Age (year)	RDA
Children to Age 10	25 - 100 mcg
Males 11 - 14	150 mcg
Males 15 - 51+	200 mcg
Females 11 - 14	150 mcg
Females 15 - 51+	180 mcg
Pregnant Women	400 mcg
Nursing Mothers	260 - 280 mcg

in malabsorption problems, cirrhosis of the liver, high alcohol intake, inflammatory bowel disease, sickle cell disease and after trauma or burns. Acute deficiency can occur in patients receiving nutrition through tubes with symptoms of diarrhea, mental irritability, depression, skin rash, alopecia and loss of taste. The signs and symptoms of deficiency and overdose of zinc and other minerals are listed in Appendix B, Table 2.

Chronic deficiency will be associated with growth retardation, alopecia, dermatitis, diarrhea, immunologic dysfunction, failure to thrive, psychological disturbances, impaired spermatogenesis and congenital malformations. Treatment with zinc sulfate results in dramatic response. Toxicity can result from excess intake, inhalation of zinc fumes by welders, intravenous administration and hemodialysis. Symptoms of acute toxicity are fever, chills, excessive gastric secretion, headache, cough, leukocytosis. Consequences of chronic toxicity can be gastric ulcer, pancreatitis, lethargy, anemia and pulmonary fibrosis with respiratory distress.

Zinc supplementation giving more than 100% of the RDA can also reduce copper status, impair immune responses, and decrease

TABLE 9.8
Best Sources of Zinc

Daily Requirement:	For Men: 15 mg RE For Women: 12 mg RE
Item	Serving
Fortified cold cereal:	2 oz
Beef, lamb, veal	3 oz
Chicken	2 legs
Oysters	3 oz.
Yogurt	2 cups

HDL cholesterol levels (Food and Nutrition Board Recommended Dietary Allowances, 1989). It is not proven that zinc cures colds and proof of safety is lacking with high doses and long-term use.

viii. Vitamin B12: Blood Booster

It is reported that over 15% of people aged 65 or older have a deficiency of Vitamin B12. If this deficiency is not treated within three to six months from the time it develops, they may suffer permanent nervous system damages. So let us tell you more about the functions of Vitamin B12:

1. Helps in the formation and regeneration of red blood cells and nerves.
2. Prevents anemia.
3. Aids in breakdown and metabolism of carbohydrates, fats and proteins
4. Maintains a healthy nervous system

TABLE 9.9

Ten Best Sources of Minerals

Mineral	Source
Calcium	Turnips, mustard greens, milk products, peas, beans
Iodine	Iodized salt, seafood, seaweed
Magnesium	Turnips, beet greens, dry beans, avocados, bananas, whole grains, green leafy vegetables
Iron	Green leafy vegetables, dry beans, dry peas, whole grains, molasses, lean meats
Zinc	Seafood, wheat, beans, dairy products, leafy vegetables, animal-derived foods
Manganese	Spinach, tea, rice, fruits
Selenium	Grains, bran, wheat germ, broccoli, clams
Chromium	Beer, beef, black pepper, vegetables
Copper	Lobster, oysters, avocados, fortified bran
Phosphorus	Grains, milk products, poultry, fish, meats, dry beans

5. Promotes growth in children
6. Increases energy
7. Helps in absorption of calcium

Deficiency consequences

What happens if you do not get enough of this vitamin? Animal products are the main sources of B12 in the diet (see Table 9.10 for other sources). Therefore, deficiency occurs frequently in vegetarians.

TABLE 9.10

Ten Best Sources of Vitamin B12

Daily Requirement:	For Men: 2 mcg RE For Women: 2 mcg RE
Item	Serving
Beef, Lamb, Pork	12 oz
Beef Liver	12 oz
Chicken Liver	2 cups
Crab, Lobster	12 oz
Catfish, Swordfish, Trout	12 oz
Mussels	12 oz
Scallops, Mackerel	12 oz
Eggs	8 oz
Skim Milk	8 cups
Yogurt	8 cups

Nutritional deficiency also occurs in chronic alcoholics. Malabsorption of Vitamin B12 also leads to deficiency in cases of stomach surgery, disease of the ileum, and failure of the pancreas.

A common cause of Vitamin B12 deficiency is pernicious anemia, which is mostly a disease of the elderly. Therefore, particularly those over age 60 should be concerned if they develop the following symptoms of pernicious anemia:

1. Symptoms related to anemia—weakness, light-headedness, ringing in ears, dizziness, palpitations.
2. Symptoms related to stomach and intestines—loss of appetite, weight loss, sore tongue.

3. Symptoms related to nervous system—numbness and tingling of extremities, weakness, loss of balance.

What should you do?

1. The ten best sources of Vitamin B12 listed in Table 9.10.
2. Do not abuse alcohol as this can lead to poor absorption of B12 from your diet.
3. Consult your doctor. He can easily make the diagnosis of pernicious anemia by blood tests. And the treatment is simple. Your doctor will give you five to six injections of 1000 mcg of B12 over a two week period followed by injections every three months. For maintenance therapy he may give you 150 mcg pills per day to be taken by mouth.

References

Cambridge heart antioxidant study. (1996) *Lancet, 347*, 781-86.

Center for Science in the Public Interest. Nutrition Action Health Center. Washington, D.C. May 1998: 3-7. Newsweek. June 7, 1993: 46-51.

Dawson-Hughes, et al. (1997). Effect of calcium and vitamin D supplementation on bone density in men and women 65 years of age and older. *New England Journal of Medicine, 337*, 670.

Diaz, M.N. (1997). Antioxidants and atherosclerotic heart disease. *New England Journal of Medicine, 337*, 408-416.

The effect of vitamin E and beta carotene on the incidence of lung cancer and other cancers in male smokers. (1994). *New England Journal of Medicine, 330*, 1029-35.

Effects of a combination of beta carotene and vitamin A on lung cancer and cardiovascular disease. (1996). *New England Journal of Medicine, 334*, 1150-1155.

Folate and vitamin B6 from diet and supplements in the relation to risk of coronary heart disease among women. (1998). *Journal of the American Medical Association, 279*, 359-364.

Food and Nutrition Board Recommended Dietary Allowances, 10th Edition. (1989). Washington, D.C.: National Academy Press

Greenberg, E.R. (1994) A clinical trial of antioxidant vitamins to prevent colorectal adenoma. *New England Journal of Medicine, 331,* 141-147.

Hunter, et al. (1993). A prospective study of the intake of vitamin C, E and A and the risk of breast cancer. *New England Journal of Medicine, 329,* 234-240.

Lack of effect of long-term supplementation with beta carotene on the incidence of malignant neoplasms and cardiovascular disease. (1996). *New England Journal of Medicine, 334,* 1145-1149.

Levine et al. (April 1999) Criteria and recommendations for vitamin C intake. *Journal of the American Medical Association, vol. 281: no. 15,* 1415.

Kushi, L.H. et al. (1996). Dietary antioxidant vitamins and death from coronary heart disease in postmenopausal women. *New England Journal of Medicine, 334,* 1156-1162.

Michell, P. (1998) *The Complete Soy Cookbook.* New York, NY: McMillan.

Rapola, J.M. et al. (1997). Randomized trial of alpha-tocopherol and beta carotene supplements on the incidence of major coronary events in men with previous myocardial infarction. *Lancet, 349,* 1715-1720.

Smith, L.H. and Wyngarden, J.B., eds. (1998). *Cecil Textbook of Medicine.* Philadelphia, PA: W.B. Saunders Co.: 1241.

Sun Sentinel Newspaper. (March 13, 1998)

Virtamoet, et al. Effect of vitamin E and beta carotene on the incidence of primary non-fatal myocardial infarction and fatal coronary heart disease. (1998). *Arch Intern. Med, 158,* 668-75.

Wolf, A. and Wolf, A.M. (December 1998). Evidence-base use of vitamin and mineral supplementation. *Hospital Medicine, 53.*

Chapter 10

❧ ❧

Ten Other "Magic Bullets" Some Good, Some Bad, Some Ugly

*"In God we trust.
All others must have data."*

– American Medical Association

In 1993, thirty-four percent of adult Americans used alternative medicine, also called complementary or integrative medicine. The most frequently used modalities were relaxation techniques, chiropractic, massage and herbs. The reasons for using alternative medicine include: dissatisfaction with conventional treatment, need for personal control and philosophical congruence. The most common symptoms for which individuals seek alternative medicine treatments are chronic pain (37%), anxiety and chronic fatigue (31% each), sprains/muscle strains (26%), addiction problems and arthritis (both 25%) and headaches (24%) [Astin, 1998]. Alternative medicine avoids an emphasis on drugs and surgery and focuses on nutrition, stress reduction and herbs.

This chapter discusses ten alternative treatments, including the use of herbs. The emphasis is on facts and evidence-based conclusions.

i. Chelation Therapy: Good-bye Bypass?

Chelation is the term that refers to the interaction of chemical substances to bind to heavy metals in the blood. The compound formed by the combination of the chelating agent and the heavy metal is water soluble, and can be excreted in the urine. The chelating agents are meant to enhance excretion of calcium and other metals such as lead, iron, copper, mercury, aluminum, cadmium and zinc. By removing calcium from the body, chelation is supposed to clean the inside of arteries where atherosclerosis plaques containing calcium line the walls of the arteries. This principle is used for patients with heart disease, circulatory problems, dizziness, memory loss, impotence and fatigue.

In the chelation process, intravenous infusions of EDTA (ethylene diamine tetra acetic acid) are given to the patient. The patient receives the infusions three times a week. Initially, 20–30 such treatments are given, and some therapists recommend six to twelve maintenance treatments per year. The cost of each treatment averages one hundred dollars.

Chelation therapy is heavily advertised in magazines and newspapers with promises of regression and reversal of heart disease. Let us look at some more promises. People with hardening of the arteries will experience an 82.5% or better improvement from chelation. In those who are prone to strokes, it can prevent strokes. Chelation is also beneficial for people with diabetes, macular degeneration, scleroderma, hypertension, arthritis, Alzheimer's disease, multiple sclerosis and high cholesterol. Besides these claims of usefulness, chelation is touted as safe, effective and inexpensive.

Despite above claims, it must be stressed that currently no evidence exists that chelation treatment is beneficial. The claims of benefits are based on uncontrolled studies. EDTA (Soffer et al, 1997) and other chelating agents are, in fact, potentially toxic and have been linked to deaths and serious medical complications. These include kidney damage, allergic reactions, drop in calcium levels, phlebitis and bleeding problems. The Medical Letter on Drug Therapy (1981) stated: "There is no acceptable evidence that chelation therapy with EDTA is effective in the treatment of arteriosclerosis, and the adverse effects of the drug can be lethal". The American Heart Association, The Food and Drug Administration (1981), The National Institutes of Health, The American Medical Association (1980), and The American College of Physicians have taken the position that there is no proven benefit of chelation therapy in the treatment of atherosclerosis, and that this therapy should not be widely used until its efficacy is established by clinical trials.

Our Advice: Chelation therapy is an unproven modality for the treatment of atherosclerosis. The claims made for its use in different other conditions are not substantiated by scientific studies. It should not be accepted as treatment for anything other than lead poisoning.

ii. DHEA: Facts and Fables

DHEA (Dehydroepiandosterone), discovered in 1934, is described as the superstar of the superhormones. It is a steroid hormone secreted by the adrenals, brain, and skin. (Whitaker and Colman, 1997). The adrenal glands produce over 150 hormones and DHEA is the most abundant hormone in the human body. Its levels are maximum at age twenty-five and may decline steadily after that (Moore, 1993).

This hormone may have a lot to do with longevity. Its low levels are associated with age related diseases such as heart disease, obesity, diabetes, cancer, osteoporosis and dementia (Rowe and Kahn, 1998). It also increases levels of insulin-like growth factor (IGF) which declines with age. Proponents of DHEA claim the following beneficial effects:

1. Improves physical and psychological well being, enhances memory, improves mood, enhances energy, relieves stress. Drops in DHEA levels cause physical and mental decline.
2. Most recent experiments show health benefits and life extension but there are no human studies. In animals it appears to reverse numerous effects associated with aging.
3. Stimulates production of immune cells, strengthens immune system and protects against bacterial and viral infections.

4. Stabilizes blood sugar, helps prevent diabetes and produces rapid remission of diabetes.
5. Has anti-cancer and anti-atherosclerosis effects (Goldberg, 1998).
6. Inhibits breast cancer in animals, and combats colon, lung and skin cancer.
7. May thin blood, lower cholesterol, and reduce risk of heart disease.
8. Shown to be definitely beneficial in lupus (Sahelian, 1996).
9. Fights obesity, and boosts sex drive.
10. Acts as an anti-aging agent in several ways: Slows the onset of coronary artery disease, prevents obesity, strengthens immune system, lowers cholesterol and combats cancer.

DHEA is not without its potential dangers. So much more needs to be learned about the actions, applications and ill effects of this powerful and all too easily available hormone (Goldberg, 1998). Significant reported side effects of DHEA included:

1. Increased IGF-1 levels with increased risk of prostate cancer
2. Liver damage
3. Acne, oily skin
4. Deepening of voice
5. Irritability
6. Mood Swings
7. Low energy level
8. Insomnia
9. Chronic fatigue and depression
10. Increased testosterone levels causing unwanted hair growth in women

Of special note: the claims of the benefits of DHEA seem to be unfounded and of dubious value because no acceptable control studies have been performed on humans. The Food and Drug Administration (FDA) and Drug Enforcement Agency (DEA) have nothing to do with DHEA. It is not currently approved for any indication by the FDA. It is a non-prescription product available in 10, 25 and 35 mg capsules. Some physicians use it to raise testosterone levels in menopausal women, in daily doses of 10–25 mg.

Our Question: If the claims of benefits of DHEA are unfounded, if there are no acceptable control studies for its use in humans, if the FDA and DEA have nothing to do with it, if it is not currently approved for any indication, and if it has been shown to cause significant side effects, why would you use it?

III. Melatonin: Miracle or Madness

Melatonin is the principal hormone secreted by the pineal gland. It is present in the blood, cerebrospinal fluid, and urine. Levels of the hormone are higher at night than in the day. The onset of darkness is a potent stimulus to melatonin release. Its production at night decreases with age. Melatonin exerts suppressive effects on many endocrine functions.

Melatonin exerts suppressive effects on many endocrine functions. Its production at night decreases with age. Melatonin has been variously described as nature's miracle hormone (Boek and Boyette, 1995), master hormone, hormone of the night and super-hormone. These impressive descriptions of the hormone go hand-in-hand with a formidable list of claims compiled by the melatonin enthusiasts. Claims indicate that melatonin:

1. Lowers total cholesterol and bad cholesterol (LDL).
2. Acts as an anti-viral agent.
3. Serves as the most powerful antioxidant.
4. Reverses aging and extends life.
5. Regulates endocrine system, stabilizes nervous system and strengthens immune system.
6. Increases resistance to cancer
7. Relieves stress. Cures jet lag.
8. Improves sex drive.
9. Prevents cataracts.
10. May prevent Alzheimer's disease and diabetes and relieve asthma.

It should be quickly added that these startling claims are still unsupported by studies on humans. Most of the claims are based on animal studies. A recent study concludes that indiscriminate use of melatonin could lead to undesirable effects and "in some circumstances melatonin may have deleterious effects on sleep" (Middleton et al., 1996). Addressing the issue of life expectancy Richard Wurtman says: "There is no evidence that melatonin has an effect on human life expectancy." (Scientific American Website, 1999). Despite the claims on behalf of Melatonin, keep in mind:

1. Very little is known about melatonin.
2. No systematic studies of possible side effects with large doses or long term use have been done; long-term safety is unknown.
3. No convincing studies of the use of melatonin for treating age-associated diseases have been done.
4. No proof is available of melatonin's beneficial effects on libido or sexual function.
5. Melatonin is contraindicated in pregnancy and breast feeding in patients with rheumatoid arthritis and lupus, if they are taking cortisones or if kidney disease is present (Levert, 1995).
6. Melatonin is not approved by the FDA.
7. Melatonin is an unregulated non-prescription product with no requirement of labels with dosages or side effects.
8. No controls for assuring purity of the product are in effect.
9. Even small doses cause headache.
10. "There is no data supporting an anti-aging effect of melatonin in humans. Uncontrolled use of melatonin to obtain anti-proliferactive and anti-aging effects is not justified." (Brzezinski, 1997).

Melatonin is sold in the form of 1 to 5 mg tablets or capsules. The advocates of melatonin recommend the following doses:

Age 40–55	1–2 mg
Age 55–65	2–3 mg
Age 65 +	3–5 mg

Our advice: Do not use melatonin without consulting your doctor. Do not accept the claims made without further acceptable studies. It may, for now, be used only as a hypnotic to promote and sustain sleep.

iv. Growth Hormone: A Gimmick?

Human growth hormone (HGH) is a protein structure that is made by the anterior pituitary gland and is released into the blood stream. During the day the circulating levels of growth hormone are very low, except after a meal or exercise when the day time levels peak. It is at night during deep sleep, that the pituitary is most active in its release of growth hormone. Once growth hormone is released, it only has a circulating life span of about 20 minutes, at which point it is cleared from the system.

Once in circulation, growth hormone produces an insulin-like effect on cells. That is, it increases the cellular uptake of carbohydrates and proteins while slowing down the degradation of fats in the body. Cells take up carbohydrates and protein to use them as energy sources for their various functions. The main purpose of the natural growth hormone is to produce growth of bones at their natural growth points and to increase muscle mass to match the growth of the bones. Once the growth hormone has been used up, the body returns to its normal functions, which means a decrease in carbohydrate uptake and a return to normal fat degradation. As we age, the levels of growth hormone produced and released by our bodies decline, mostly due to the decreased rate of growth that comes with age (Katzung, 1998).

In the past few years there have been many claims of the fantastic changes that occur in people who have been receiving intramuscular dosages of Human Growth Hormone. Accordingly HGH is the new "miracle drug" of the 20th century. Listed below are ten of the most common claims to the benefits of HGH therapy:

1. Restoration of muscle mass without exercise, increased strength and stamina.
2. Restoration of lost hair.
3. Decrease of body fat without exercise or diet modifications, youthful appearance.
4. Increased sexual function.
5. Restoration of the sizes of the liver, pancreas, heart and other organs that shrink with age.

6. Improved vision.
7. Improved immune function.
8. Elevation of mood, increased mental alertness, improved sleep, increased memory retention.
9. Younger, tighter skin with removal of wrinkles, stronger bones.
10. Removal of cellulite.

All of these claims sound wonderful, especially in a society like ours where we are always looking for the quick and easy fix to the effects of aging. But it should be noted that none of these claims has been supported by any significant scientific studies.

What the people advocating all of these wonderful claims don't tell you about are the following ten possible increased risks associated with HGH therapy (Dorman, 1998 and Seidman, 1997):

1. Cancer of prostate
2. Low blood pressure
3. Uncontrolled bleeding
4. Leukemia in children
5. Congestive heart disease
6. Carpal tunnel syndrome, arthritis
7. Disturbances of the gastrointestinal system
8. Edema of legs
9. Gynecomastia (the development of large and tender breasts in men)
10. Resistance to insulin

These are rather serious side effects. In no way are the benefits of reversal of a few cosmetic signs of aging outweighed by the risk of getting cancer or heart disease. Even the most minor sounding of these side effects has significant consequences.

The human growth hormone is "pushed" mainly as an anti-aging remedy. Searching for the fountain of youth, Susan V. Seligson went to a Las Vegas Clinic as a patient to get "untested" human growth hormone injections for $17,302 a year. In the end she wrote, "Even if I had $20,000 to spare, I'd rather treat my mind and body to a trip around the world" (Seligson, 1998).

The Food and Drug Administration has only approved Human Growth Hormone injections for the treatment of physically stunted children and AIDS patients who suffer from severe wasting of the body.

Our Conclusion: Due to all of the unknown factors and serious side effects of Human Growth Hormone therapy, do not use it as a youth elixir until further studies prove its worth.

v. Glutathione: Good or Bad?

Glutathione is a naturally occurring compound in plants and animals that has been called a "superstar" of longevity research. But can it really help delay aging?

Glutathione, also known as glutathione peroxidase, is an antioxidant, which partly blocks damage to the cell's DNA that accumulates with age. By virtue of this action, the process of natural deterioration of the body is slowed. This damage is believed to be a major factor, not only in general signs of aging, but also in conditions such as cancer, heart disease, Parkinson's disease, and cerebral vascular degeneration.

Several claims have been made about the actions of glutathione. It is reported to boost immunity; break up fats before they do damage; prevent and cure some forms of Type II diabetes; prevent macular degeneration, an eye disease that affects the elderly; prevent lung problems; and keep blood cholesterol from becoming oxidized (Carper, 1995).

While the body makes glutathione naturally, production decreases with age. In fact, the glutathione levels drop about 17% from age 40–60. You can add it to your bloodstream most effectively by eating fresh or frozen raw fruits and vegetables, as opposed to canned or cooked varieties. Avocado, watermelon, asparagus, grapefruit, acorn squash, strawberries, potatoes, tomatoes and broccoli are good sources of glutathione. So are walnuts and fresh meats. Glutathione is sold in the form of powders and tablets. A daily dose of 25–50 mg is adequate. This amount can easily be obtained from fruits and vegetables.

Our advice: Since glutathione is present in healthy foods, supplements are unnecessary if you eat a nutritious diet. Consult your physician before you take glutathione, especially if you are ill.

vi. Coenzyme Q–10: Does it Rev Up the Cells?

Coenzyme Q–10 is one of the antioxidant supplements most often used by athletes (Cooper, 1994). Believed to help reverse age-related deterioration of vital organs, this enzyme helps put more pep in your step as the years go by. It's all the rage among people who want to live longer.

Coenzyme Q–10, or ubiquinol–10, is a natural substance found in the body. An antioxidant, it prevents damage by free radicals. Beyond that, some researchers consider CoQ–10 the "spark" that starts off cells on their vital processes. Without it, the theory goes, life cannot go on.

CoQ–10 is thought to be particularly useful to heart muscles, which require an extraordinary amount of energy to do work. There are also claims of CoQ–10 protecting against atherosclerosis, lowering blood pressure and protecting the brain from degenerative diseases. Immune system function may also be enhanced.

As with glutathione, CoQ–10 production lags with age. You can replenish your supply through foods such as fatty fish, liver and kidney, beef, soy oil and peanuts. Thirty milligrams is a good daily dose for healthy people. Supplements of vitamin E, selenium and B vitamins also help your body produce CoQ–10. No tests are available to quantify CoQ–10.

Our advice: While the outlook on CoQ–10 is promising, its antioxidant cousin vitamin E performs many of the same functions and also stimulates production of CoQ–10. Supplements do not appear necessary, particularly if you eat a balanced diet.

vii. Ginseng: Chinese Cure–All Herb?

Ginseng belongs to the genus "panax" from the Latin word "panacea," or "cure-all." And while it may not be able to do quite everything it is reputed to, it sells well (Hyla, 1999). In the U. S., ginseng is the top-selling herbal product. Americans spend $78 million yearly on ginseng. It is available in the form of tonics, slices, powders, tablets, extracts, confections, fruit, and mineral drinks.

Ginseng increases resistance to stress and enhances mental functions, stamina, and immunity. In this capacity, it has been used by Russian Olympic athletes to improve performance and by ordinary workers throughout the world to decrease illness during work days.

Ginseng takes three forms: Panax ginseng (China, Korea, Japan and Russia), Panax quinquefolia (North America) and Eleutherococcus senticosus (Siberia), which is technically not a ginseng at all but functions in a similar way. The ginseng root is the source of the herb's benefits, which are legendary. Ginseng is a tonic that is considered to increase the body's resistance to disease, increase stamina and enhance recovery (Howe, 1996). For cancer patients, it is thought to ease side effects of radiation, protect normal cells against the harmful effects of radiation, and stimulate the production of white blood cells. For people with diabetes, the claim is that it helps enhance production of insulin and lower blood sugar. Those with high cholesterol have been reported to benefit from its ability to lower bad cholesterol (LDL) and raise good cholesterol (HDL). The elderly and frail appreciate its stimulant effect. It is reported that many people with a low sex drive benefit from the aphrodisiac qualities of the American and Korean varieties.

Other reported uses include treatment of absentmindedness, alcoholism (hangovers), anemia, asthma, boils, bronchitis, bruises, convulsions, coughing, dizziness, dysentery, dysmenorrhea, eating disorders, gas, gout, hardening of the arteries, headache, insomnia, kidney disease, nausea, general pain, and vertigo.

The recommended dose is two 100 mg capsules daily containing four percent ginsanosides or 10–30 drops of tincture or extract.

Ginseng can cause allergic reactions. Panax ginseng may cause menstrual abnormalities, breast tenderness, as well as high blood pressure. Chinese herbalists warn against its use in acute inflammatory disease and bronchitis due to its stimulating tendencies. As with most herbal remedies, check with your doctor before using it especially if you are pregnant or nursing. Ginseng has been implicated as a cause of decreased response to Warfarin.

Our advice: For simple ailments, ginseng is safe and may prove effective in increasing the sense of well-being. In the case of more serious conditions, seek medical advice before using it. The Federal Bureau of Alcohol, Tobacco and Firearms warns that some ginseng products may contain a high concentration of alcohol.

viii. Gingko: Another Memory Booster?

The North Americans have just recently come to appreciate the beneficial effects of "the smart herb." The publicity of these herbs ushered yearly sales of gingko to $66 million. The Chinese relied on gingko as early as 2800 B.C. to restore memory. What's more, they have used the fruit and leaves of the ancient gingko biloba or maidenhair tree to alleviate many other problems associated with aging, from brain disorders to clogged arteries, "thick" blood, metabolic dysfunction and inadequate irrigation of tissues. In addition, gingko makes quick work of free radicals. These are the molecules or molecule fragments that cause cells to break down, thus hastening the aging process. By utilizing them before they can cause significant damage, the aging process can be slowed.

The gingko tree is the last of a species of plants known as ginkgoales, which date back more than 200 million years. Most of the trees were destroyed after the Jurassic period, but some apparently survived in east Asia. At present, most if not all of the known gingko trees are found in Asia and exist in cultivation.

The wide-ranging benefits, which can be grouped into neurological, cardiovascular, and metabolic effects, are in fact related. Gingko improves circulation to many parts of the body, including the brain. It may improve mental function in patients with dementia by enhancing blood flow to the brain. Today, studies are underway to determine its use in reversing some of the effects of Alzheimer's disease. It must be emphasized that clinical trials to study gingko are small and poorly designed.

In addition to those listed above, gingko's uses include: treatment of skin and eye damage caused by ultraviolet rays; asthma, impotence, vertigo, headache, tinnitus, partial deafness, Raynaud's syndrome, diabetic tissue damage when there is danger of gangrene, anxiety, depression, complications of stroke and skull injuries, hair loss and premenstrual syndrome.

Europeans are quite convinced of gingko's powers. Preparations based on its leaves are used for therapy of peripheral vascular, cerebrovascular conditions and disturbances of brain function. Their popularity makes it a half-billion-dollar business. In Germany in particular, a four-month study of the long-term effects on vigilance and mental performance, published in 1992, tested 72 outpatients at three test centers. Short-term memory improved after six weeks, while the subjects' learning rate was enhanced after just four months. They concluded gingko improves short-term memory and learning ability.

Gingko has been associated with certain side effects. It has been reported to cause spontaneous bleeding and produce rare cases of mild gastrointestinal problems, headaches and skin allergies.

Our advice: Do not take gingko biloba if you are taking aspirin, Ticlid, Plavix or Persantine. Note that the purity and potency of gingko extracts sold in the U.S. are unknown, and therefore the effects may be variable

ix. Ginger: Grabbing the Spotlight

For most of us, the word "ginger" brings to mind lifelong memories of ginger snaps, gingerbread and ginger ale. But in fact, ginger has as honored a place in the medicine cabinet as it does in the kitchen.

Ginger, or zingiber officinale, is a reedlike plant, native to the East Indies, but now grown in most tropical countries. Pungent and spicy, it belongs to the same plant family as its slightly more exotic cousins cardamon and turmeric.

Humans have benefited from the medicinal properties of ginger for thousands of years. The Greeks and Indians used it to enhance digestion. Egyptians believed that it prevented infectious epidemics. To improve the cardiovascular system and relieve colds, the Chinese added it to tonics. Hawaiians poured it into shampoos and massage oils. And the Romans considered ginger an essential and highly effective aphrodisiac.

Throughout the world, the medical claims for ginger span a wide variety of ailments, in large part due to its anti-histamine and anti-inflammatory qualities. Medical anthropologist John Heinerman (1993) showed that ginger root works wonders for morning sickness and nausea accompanying the premenstrual syndrome. A daily "dose" of fresh, uncooked ginger can lessen the severity and frequency of migraines.

Ginger has also been used for alcoholism, angina, poor appetite, arthritis, broken bones, catarrh (mucus), chills and colds, colic, cramps, diarrhea, digestive disorders, fevers, flu, impotence, infectious disease prevention, memory problems, muscle aches, rheumatism, sinusitis, sprain and tonsillitis.

Our advice: Since ginger has no significant side effects and an abundance of uses, keep some on hand, either fresh, powdered or in liquid extract form. As with most remedies, consult a physician before taking large amounts while ill or pregnant.

x. Garlic: Wards Off Vampires *and* Helps Your Heart

"Five things have been said about garlic: it assuages hunger, warms the body, brings joy, increases virility and destroys intestinal lice. There are those who say it engenders love and dispels envy."

–Babylonian Talmud: Baba Kama

One day Mahatma Gandhi told A.F.'s father: "Eat two garlics, one onion and one tomato every day and you will live to be 100." If you thought smell was the only area in which garlic is strong, take a look at ten things you may not know about this familiar and unusually powerful vegetable.

1. Allium sativum, or garlic, is a member of the amaryllis family. The ancient Egyptians worshipped it. The Greek Olympians used

is to keep them strong. And as any fan of Dracula can attest, it was believed to keep vampires at bay in the Middle Ages.
2. More than a dozen studies have revealed garlic's role in reducing cholesterol. In a British experiment, a 12% reduction in cholesterol was evident after just four weeks of treatment. Similar results were revealed in German research with more than 250 patients. After twelve weeks of garlic consumption, subjects' serum cholesterol level plunged by 12%, while triglycerides dropped by 17% compared to the control group.
3. As another boon to the heart, garlic is known to reduce blood pressure and generally enhance the cardiovascular system.
4. Garlic has long been considered a powerful aphrodisiac and treatment for impotence. Not only does it enhance blood flow, it also contains an enzyme called nitric oxide synthase that is involved in the mechanism of erection!
5. Research carried out in Britain has revealed that pregnant women who eat garlic have a lower risk of pre-eclampsia.
6. Garlic contains over a dozen antioxidants. A recent study in Pennsylvania revealed that injections of diallyl disulphide, a compound found in cut or crushed raw garlic, can prevent cancer-causing agents from binding to human breast cells. Other research indicates that garlic both prevents and treats a variety of cancers.
7. Garlic is a potent antibiotic. Since many believe that heart disease is caused by an infection, this helps explain its heart-healing powers.
8. Garlic loses its antibiotic properties when it is cooked or dried. Unfortunately garlic capsules do not have the full strength of fresh, raw garlic either. If you're concerned about your breath, chew a sprig of parsley after eating garlic.
9. Garlic is good for anxiety, stress and depression.
10. Recommended dosage: Half to two cloves each day can lower blood sugar. So avoid it if you are hypoglycemic. More than three garlic cloves a day may cause diarrhea, gaseousness, bloating and fever.

Summary

Our discussions of the alternative treatments indicate that some of them are safe and others are not. In 1997 consumers spent more than $12 billion on natural supplements (Greenwald, 1998). Some 629 million visits are made by Americans to alternative healthcare providers and only 386 million visits to see their primary care physicians. Herbs can heal but they can hurt too. Physicians have legitimate concerns about their safety and efficacy, and so should you. If you are planning to use herbs and other alternative treatments remember the following:

1. "Natural" does not mean it is safe.
2. Herbal medicines are not required to be tested for safety.
3. Some products may be contaminated; make sure the product you are using is pure .
4. Look for standardized preparations.
5. Purchase products from reputable companies that do research.
6. Herbal products may make certain medical problems worse.
7. Always inform your physician what you are taking.
8. The American Academy of Family Physicians recommends that you talk with your physician before using herbal products if you have any of the following ten conditions: high blood pressure, diabetes mellitus, thyroid problem, psychiatric problem, enlarged prostate gland, blood clotting problems, epilepsy, glaucoma, stroke, Parkinson's disease.
9. Don't develop a false sense of security and ignore serious problems because you have herbal protection.
10. Don't sacrifice healthy life-styles thinking that herbs will do it all.

References

American Medical Association Dept. of Drugs. (1998). *AMA Drug Evaluations*. (4th edition). Chicago, 1998: 902-3.

Astin, J.A. (1998). Why patients use alternative medicine. Results of a national study. *Journal of the American Medical Association, 279*, 1548.

Boek, S.J. and Boyette, M. (1995). *Nature's Miracle Hormone, the Melatonin Way*. New York, NY: A. Lynn Sonberg Books.

Brzezinski, A. (1997). Melatonin in humans. *New England Journal of Medicine, 336*, 186-95.

Carper, J. (1995). *Stop Aging Now!* New York, N.Y: Harper Collins, 124-135.

Colman, C. and Whitaker, J. (1993). *Shed Ten Years in Ten Weeks*. New York, NY: Simon and Schuster.

Cooper, K.H. (1994). *Dr. Kenneth H Cooper's Antioxidant Revolution*. Nashville, TN: Thomas Nelson, 72.

Dorman, L.E. (1998, Spring). *Growth Hormone Therapy*. Paper presented at the meeting of The American College for Advancement of Medicine, Fort Lauderdale, FL.

EDTA. (1981). Chelation therapy for arteriosclerotic heart disease. *Medical Letter Drug Therapy, 23*, 51.

Greenwald, J.(1998, Nov. 23). Herbal Healing. *Time*.

Heinerman, J. (1993). *Healing Power of Herbs*. Boca Raton, FL: Globe Publications, 43-45.

Howe, M. (1996). The Chinese Medicine Chest. *Living Country Living, 19*, 16.

Hyla, C. (1999). *All About Herbs*. Garden City Park, New York, N.Y: Garden City Park, 41-46.

Kahn, R.L. and Rowe, J.W. (1998). *Successful Aging*. NY, NY: Pantheon Books.

Katzung, B.F. (1998). *Basic and Clinical Pharmacology.* (7th Edition). Stamford, CT: Appleton and Lange.

Levert, S. (1995). *Melatonin. The Anti-Aging Hormone.* New York, NY: Avon Books.

Middleton, B.A. et al. (1996). Fragmented sleep patterns. *Lancet, 348,* 9026.

Moore, T.J. (1993). *Lifespan. Who Lives Longer and Why.* New York, NY: Simon and Schuster.

Seidman, D. (1997). *The Longevity Sourcebook.* Los Angeles, CA: Lowell House.

Seligson, S.V. (1998, May). Antiaging. *Hippocrates,* 45.

Soffer, A. et al. (1964). *Chelation Therapy.* Springfield, IL: Charles C. Thomas.

Wurtman, R. (1999). Explorations—Melatonin mania. *Scientific American.* Website: http://www.sciam.com.

Section IV.

Exercise

Chapter 11

Exercise: Ten Best Ways

A report of the Surgeon General in 1996 indicated clearly that regular physical activity reduces the risk for coronary heart disease, diabetes, colon cancer, and several other major chronic diseases and conditions. It is also clear that 30 minutes of daily moderate physical activity yields substantial health benefits. "Some activity is better than none, more is better than some, until at one point it is possible to do too much" (Pratt, 1999).

In this chapter, the ten best exercises and their benefits are listed, followed by the discussion of walking, running and stretching in subsequent chapters. See Table 11.1 for comparative calorie expenditure for each of the exercises.

Ten Best Exercises

1. Walking—good for all ages. The absolute best.
2. Swimming—harmless, painless, good for all the parts of the body. And, you don't have to know how to swim.
3. Running—great, if you're generally fit.
4. Cycling—easy, relaxing, effortless if you want to make it.
5. Tennis—one of the best sports for exercise, if you are fit.
6. Golf—entertaining, challenging, relaxing. Don't use the cart.
7. Dancing—the ultimate pleasure, but don't drink alcohol.
8. Aerobic—on indoor machines, if weather is against you.
9. Bowling—exercise with social fun.
10. Hiking, skating, skiing, if you can.

TABLE 11.1
Energy Expenditures for 160 lb Person

Activity	Calories burned per hour
Aerobic Dancing	500
Basketball	556
Cycling (12 mph)	410
Golf	308
Lawn Mowing	500
Roller Skating	432
Running/Jogging (10 mph)	1280
Swimming (50 yard/minute)	500
Tennis (Singles)	400
Walking (4½ mph)	500

Ten Health Benefits of Exercise

1. Exercise burns calories and helps you lose weight.
2. Lowers blood pressure, increases HDL cholesterol, decreases LDL cholesterol and risk of heart attack, stroke, cancer, and diabetes.
3. Helps you eat less and controls appetite.
4. Builds muscles and muscle strength, burns fat.
5. Increases metabolic rate, metabolism, and heart's efficiency.
6. Helps keep weight down and maintains healthy weight.
7. Improves mental acuity and promotes thought process.
8. Helps you sleep better.
9. Relieves stress and tensions.
10. Makes you feel good mentally and physically and prolongs life.

Ten Ways To Beat Exercise Burnout

Has your get-up-and-go for exercise gone? You may be suffering from exercise burnout. In some ways it's similar to the garden-variety burnout we all suffer when we've worked too hard. Boredom. Fatigue. Perhaps, a bit of depression. If your workout has gotten repetitive, you're sure to benefit from these ten ways to beat exercise burnout:

1. Try a new exercise you've never done before.
2. Do a new variation on an old exercise, such as using Nautilus instead of free weights.
3. Mix and match exercise routines.
4. Find a buddy to keep you company-and to get you going.
5. Set goals, such as ten more laps of swimming.
6. Buy yourself new equipment.
7. Get a heart rate monitor. The challenge: Staying within that all-important specific heart rate zone.
8. Change gyms or go to a new park to jog.
9. Buy yourself new workout gear.
10. Add music to your routine, or change present tunes.

References

American Heart Association. (1996). *Statement on Exercise: Benefits and Recommendations for Physical Activity Programs for All Americans.* Website: http://www.amhrt.org.

Pratt, M. (1999). Benefits of lifestyle activity vs. structured exercise. *Journal of the American Medical Association, 281, 4*, 375-376.

Chapter 12

Stretching

The Great Yawn Stretch

Do you yawn? Yes, you do. Who doesn't? Yawning is nature's way of making you stretch. Analyze a whole yawning act and you will realize that it involves many acts of stretching. First, your mouth opens against resistance and then relaxes, often stretching your facial muscles. Second, with every yawn the chest expands fully with deep inhalation stretching your chest muscles, and then relaxing them with a short exhalation. As you do this, your shoulders move up and down, stretching more muscles. Third, you naturally stretch your arms up and out and sometimes interlock your fingers at the back of the neck. This stretches many more muscles. Thus, yawning is a beautiful act of natural stretching.

In this section we will first explain the principles of stretching, the benefits, and the limitations of stretching. This will be followed by various stretching techniques. The techniques are carefully selected to fit the needs of people of all ages, ones that can be performed at any place in different general circumstances and environments. You will find a variety of stretching exercises described here. Select and use the ones that best suit your needs and physical conditions. For special circumstances and for more elaborate information, the reader is referred to the books on stretching: *The Book About Stretching* by Sven A. Sölveborn; *Stretch and Strengthen* by Judy Alter; and *The Complete Idiot's Guide to Health Stretching* by Chris Verna and Steve Hosid.

Basic Principles of Stretching Before Workout or Sport

1. Warm-up first
2. After a static muscle contraction against resistance, relax and then stretch the muscle.
3. Start slowly and increase ability gradually.
4. Relax and carry out sustained stretch.
5. Think about the exercise you will be doing and then focus attention on the muscles to be stretched.
6. Do not stretch to the point of pain.
7. Stretch on a regular basis.
8. Alternate muscle groups being stretched.
9. Cool-down towards end of stretching.
10. If stretching is performed for injury or illness rehabilitation or if you are experiencing pain, consult your physician before trying any of the stretches.

Ten Benefits of Stretching

Many people believe that stretching is a prelude to a more intense workout. We believe that it is much more than that. For the general population it is an excellent relaxation activity that promotes health and fitness. The benefits of stretching include the following:

1. Increased metabolism in the muscles and other soft tissues and increased flexibility. Increased flexibility creates better work conditions for the muscles, tendons and bones.
2. Greater muscle power.
3. Increased strength, speed, agility, balance, and greater precision.
4. Decreased muscle soreness after workouts or sporting activities.
5. Decreased incidence of muscle pulls, muscle tears and overuse injuries.
6. Improved stamina and performance.
7. Decreased stress.
8. Quicker recovery from the effects of injury and illnesses.
9. Greater mental and physical relaxation.
10. Better health and improved longevity.

When to Stretch

1. Right after you wake up.
2. Before workouts or sports.
3. Before exercises such as walking, jogging, swimming.
4. During coffee breaks.
5. During the interval at movies.
6. Between classes at school, college.
7. At your computer or typewriter or with sedentary jobs, every hour.
8. During examinations and in libraries.
9. When recovering from injuries or illness.
10. Before going to bed. Essentially, all the time.

Where to Stretch

1. In bed, upon waking.
2. At home, if you are not working.
3. At work, why not?
4. On the street or in the park.
5. In a gymnasium or on a playground.
6. In a hotel room if you are traveling.
7. At school, between classes.
8. During a long trip, whether on a plane, car or train.
9. While standing in line.
10. While talking on the phone or watching television. In fact, everywhere.

Ten Best Stretching Exercises In Bed

1. Lie flat with your back in contact with the mattress, palms down, and fingers stretched. Rhythmically and alternatively move the entire upper extremity with your shoulders up and down, as far as you can, not too fast, not too slow. Do this ten times. This will stretch and relax your muscles between the shoulders and the neck and the muscles between the shoulder blades in the back.

2. Lie flat with your back in contact with the mattress, palms down and fingers stretched. Rhythmically and alternatively move the entire lower extremities up and down as far as you can, not too fast, not too slow. Do this ten times. This will stretch and relax your muscles in your back on the sides of the spine.
3. Hyperextend and hyperflex alternatively your feet at the ankles to their full extent. Do this ten times. This will stretch and relax your leg muscles.
4. Hyperflex and straighten out your elbows to their full extent, simultaneously ten times. This is great for your biceps muscles.
5. Turn your neck fully to the right and then to the left ten times to stretch and relax the neck muscles.
6. Fully flex and extend your legs at the knees ten times to loosen up the thigh and leg muscles.
7. Fully flex and extend your thighs (with flexed knees and bring one knee to your chest, hold the knee with both hands and pull in gently). Alternate legs and do this ten times.
8. Sit up by the side of the bed with your feet touching the floor, hyperextend and hyperflex your neck alternatively ten times.
9. While seated as above, stretch your arms completely to the sides and rotate the shoulders and the torso to and fro as far as you can.
10. Take a long deep breath in and exhale fully. Do this ten times. Now you are prepared for further workouts and stretch.

Prescription

To feel relaxed and energized, stretch in bed every morning at home or elsewhere.

Ten Stretching Exercises for Executives: No Equipment Needed

1. Jumping Jacks: Stand erect with feet together and arms at the side. Swing the arms upwards until they come above the head and spread the feet apart simultaneously. In second movement bring the arms to the side and feet together as in the starting position (Diagram 2). Do this ten times.

2. Trunk Rotation: Stand erect. Raise your arms to shoulder level. With your feet slightly separated, twist your trunk and arms to one side without lifting your heels. Twist five times to one side and then five times to the other side. This will stretch muscles of the back, sides and shoulder (Diagram 3).
3. Shoulder Stretches with arm circles and toe raises: Stand erect with the feet about a foot apart and arms stretched to sides. Swing arms upward and around making big circles. Raise arms and cross overhead and as you do this raise your feet. Do this ten times (Diagram 4).
4. Extremities Stretch: Sit on your chair with your back straight up. Extend your arms and legs straight out in front of you. Raise your arms straight and at the same time separate your legs about 18 inches. Keep them stretched for a few seconds. Then, bring the arms down and legs together keeping them straight out in front. Now flex and extend your feet for a few seconds. Repeat this exercise ten times.
5. Chest Stretch: Stand straight in a corner of the room facing the wall and feet about 12 inches apart. Put your hands against the walls and push your chest forwards to feel tightening of the chest. Do this ten times. Then put the forearms against the walls and push the chest forwards. Repeat this ten times.
6. Calf Stretch: Stand erect and then lean against a wall with hands at chest level. Slide your right leg backward about two feet and flex the left knee. Lean your whole body forward to stretch the right leg. Maintain this stretch for ten seconds. Repeat the process on the opposite side for ten seconds (Diagram 5).
7. Side stretch: Stand erect with one arm extended upwards and the other on the side of the body. Keep feet apart about the width of your shoulders. With feet flat, bend your torso to the right with the left arm stretching overhead. Return to the starting position. Repeat five times. Use same procedure five times for the other side. This will stretch medial muscles of the thigh and the lateral muscles of the torso (Diagram 6).

Stretching 153

8. Thigh and Hip Muscles Stretch: Stand on your right leg facing a wall with your left hand against the wall and your left knee flexed fully. Hold onto the left foot with your right hand and pull the foot backwards and upwards as much as possible to bring the left heel close to the left buttock. Maintain this position for ten seconds. Bring left arm and left leg down and relax. Repeat the process with the opposite side for ten seconds.
9. Shoulder and Chest Stretch: Stand erect with your arms at shoulder level and elbows bent. Force your elbows backwards slowly and bring them back to the starting position. Repeat this ten times (Diagram 7).
10. Front leg stretch: Sit on the floor with one leg extended straightforward. Bend the other leg at the knee to bring the sole touching the inner aspect of the thigh of the extended leg. Bend forwards as much as possible to bring the head to touch the knee of the extended leg. Stretch five times. Repeat five times with the opposite leg (Diagram 8).

Additional Good Stretches

It is not possible to do some stretches in bed or in the office. These are grouped below to complete the stretching of most of the muscles in the body.

Legs and Buttocks Stretching

Stand erect with hands on the hips. Bend forwards slowly to about 90-degree angle (Diagram 9). Return slowly to starting position. Repeat this several times.

Hamstring Stretches

Sit on a floor. Keep one leg extended straight forward. Place the other leg forward with bent knee so that the sole of the foot is in contact with the inner aspect of the thigh of the extended leg (Diagram 10).

Bend forward and make the head touch the knee. Stay in this position for 20 seconds, then relax. Repeat the procedure with the other leg.

Groin Stretch

Sit on the floor with knees bent forwards and the soles of feet touching each other in the front. Grasp the knees and press them down sideways at the same time pulling the upper body forwards as close to the feet as possible and hold for 20 seconds (Diagram 11). Repeat a few times.

Lower Back Stretching

This helps stretch the muscles in the lower back and buttocks. To do this lie on your back on the floor with your legs extended. Then lift and bend one leg with full flexion of the knee. Pull the knee towards the chest with your hands. Keep the opposite leg flat on the surface. Do this a few times. Repeat the same process with the opposite leg a few times (Diagram 12).

Sit-up Stretching

This stretching strengthens the abdominal and hip flexor muscles. To do this lie flat on the floor with knees flexed and hands clasped behind the neck. Raise the head and the trunk to an upright position, then return to starting position. Repeat this several times. (Diagram 13).

References

Alter, J. (1986). *Stretch and Strengthen.* Boston, MA: Houston Mifflin, Co.

Hosid, S. and Verna, C. (1998). *The Complete Idiot's Guide to Health Stretching.* New York, NY: Alpha Books.

Sölveborn, S.A. (1985). *The Book About Stretching.* Japan: Japan Publications, Inc.

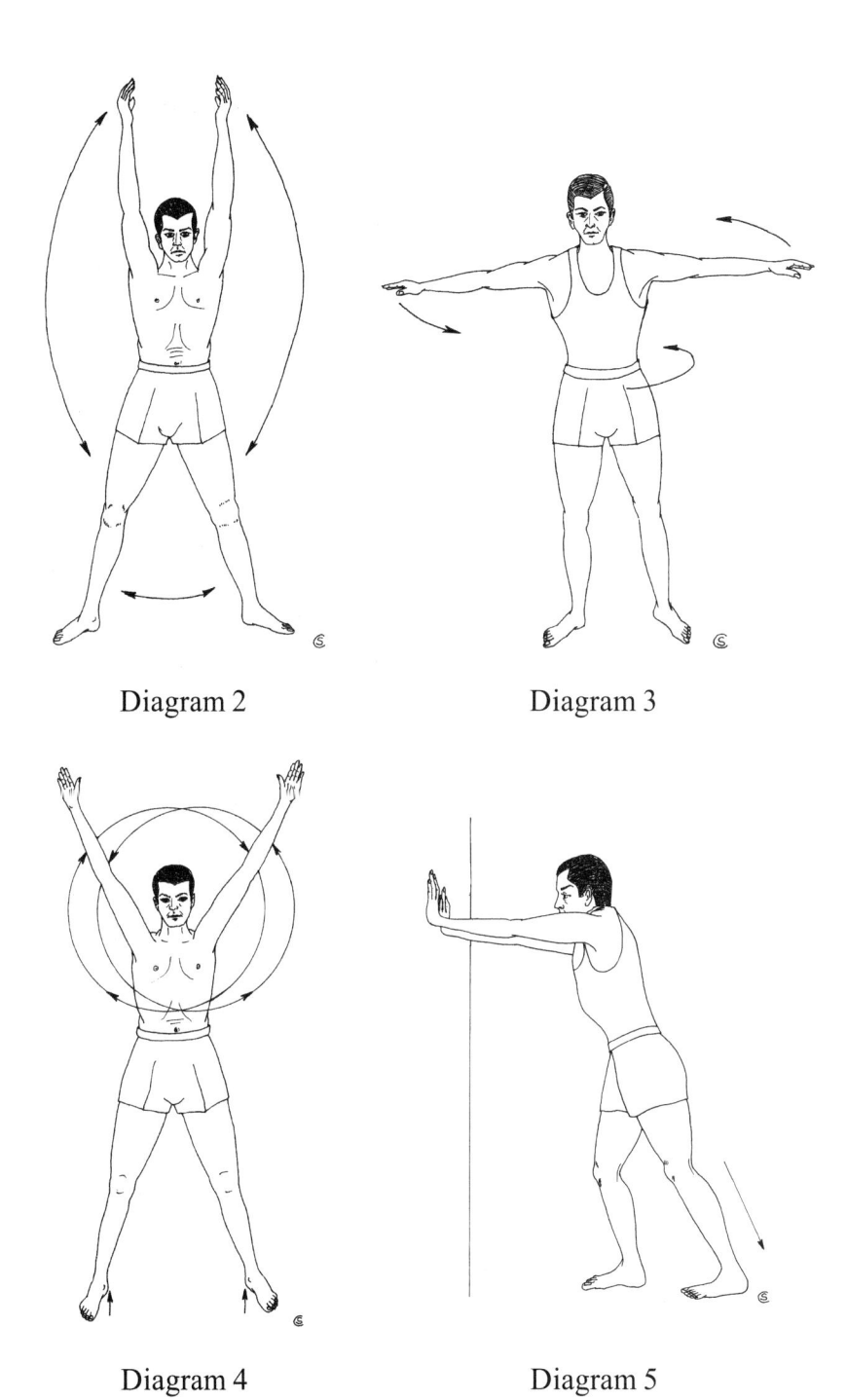

Stretching 155

Diagram 2

Diagram 3

Diagram 4

Diagram 5

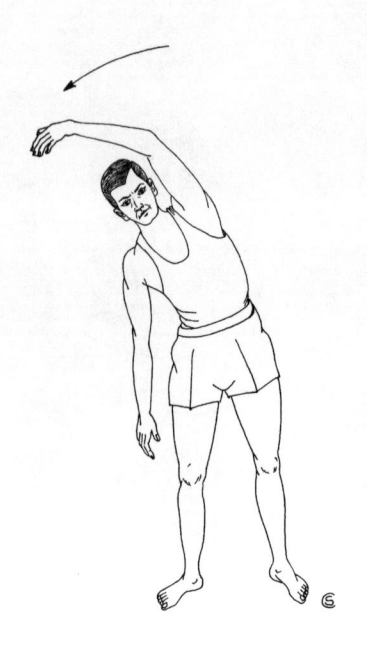

Diagram 6

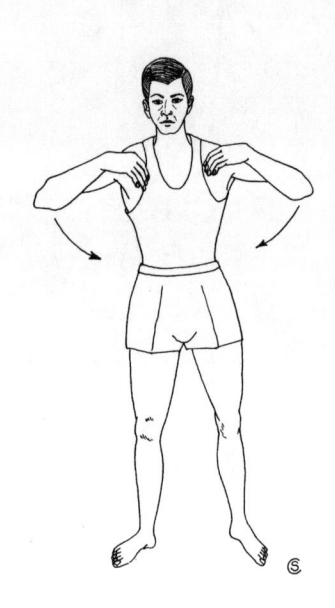

Diagram 7

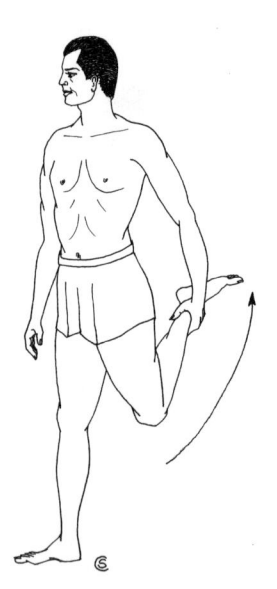

Diagram 8

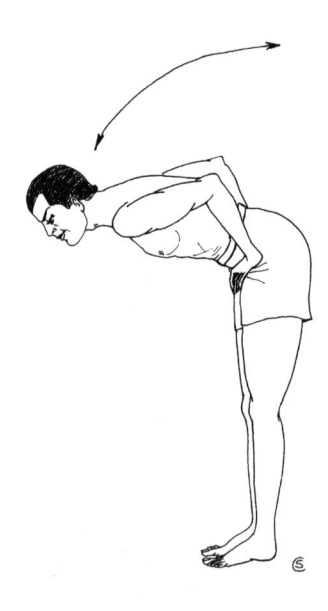

Diagram 9

Stretching 157

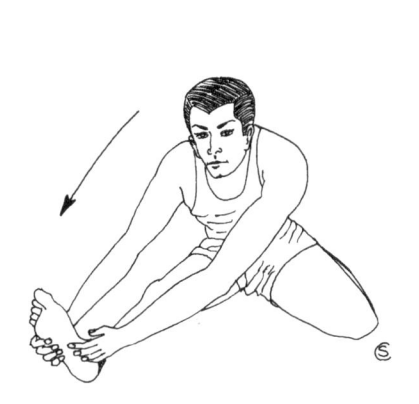

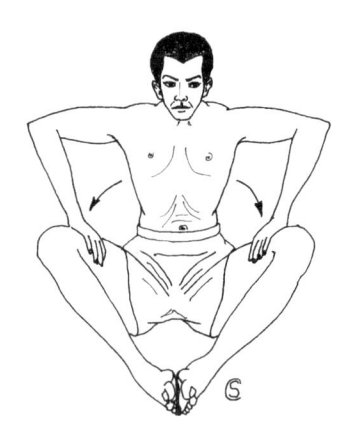

Diagram 10

Diagram 11

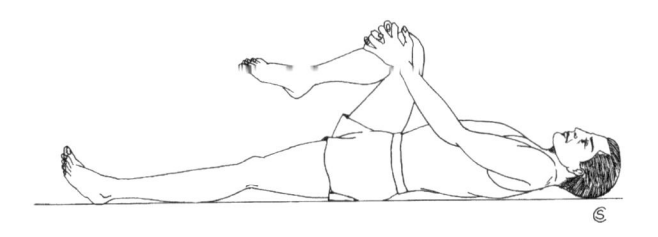

Diagram 12

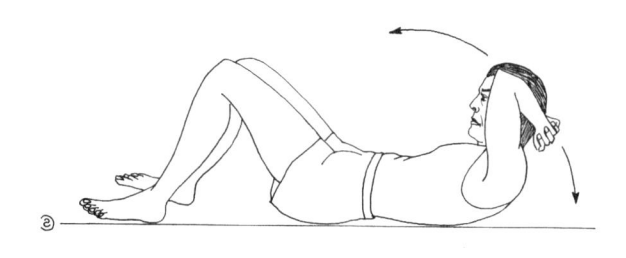

Diagram 13

Chapter 13

Walking

"The Sovereign invigorator of the body is exercise, and of all exercises walking is the best."

–Thomas Jefferson

Benefits of Walking

Walking is the perfect exercise because it is inexpensive, effortless, easy, joyful, thought provoking and health promoting. That is why Hippocrates said: "Walking is man's best medicine." The physiologic benefits of walking are (Stutman with Africano, 1980)

1. Improves heart function.
2. Lowers blood pressure. Reduces high blood pressure.
3. Improves efficiency and capacity.
4. Increases energy level.
5. Reduces risk of clot formation.
6. Relaxes and reduces tension, anxiety, and tension headaches. Improves self image and self esteem. Quickens thought process. Prevents depression.
7. Lowers cholesterol and triglycerides level, increases level of good cholesterol and reduces risk of heart attacks and strokes.

8. Decreases appetite. Improves digestion.
9. Helps weight control. Increases general fitness.
10. Increases longevity.

If walking has so many benefits and if it is man's best medicine, why not get ready and go. Wear appropriate clothes and shoes. Shoes are a very important part of walking. Choose them wisely. Here are ten features the shoes should have (Malkin, 1995):

1. Comfort.
2. Lots of toe room.
3. Flexible at the ball of the foot.
4. Well cushioned.
5. Firm heel support.
6. Achilles notch at the back of shoe.
7. Appropriate added padding for foot arch support.
8. Good traction pattern on the bottom of sole.
9. Slightly convex, not flat, sole.
10. Flexible upper part of shoe.

When you come back from your walk and don't feel like removing your shoes, it means you have good shoes.

Right Ways to Walk

"Few people know how to take a walk. The qualifications are...endurance, plain clothes, good old shoes, an eye for nature, good humor, vast curiosity, good speech, good silence and nothing too much."

– Ralph Waldo Emerson

Walking Right Physically

You have the right clothes on and the best shoes you can buy. You are ready to go. But before you take off, here are some tips on walking the right way (Malkin, 1995).

1. Keep feet parallel.
2. Let the inside edge of each foot fall on the same line.
3. Obtain optimum stride by hip advancement.
4. Contract heel first.
5. Bring leg forward easily and comfortably.
6. Keep posture relaxed with forward, upward motion.
7. Let pelvis and chest lead keep shoulders relaxed.
8. Bend elbows 90°, swing arms back and forth and move hands forward to mid-chest.
9. Keep hip movement flexible and advance hips directly forwards
10. Pace in an unstrained way.

Finally walk as fast as you comfortably can.

Walking Safety Tips

Right shoes, right ways to walk, now let us look at the ten ways to walk with safety in mind (Meyers, 1992):

1. Walk defensively.
2. Look both ways before crossing the street.
3. Stay on the outside of a blind curve.
4. Walk on shoulders or foot paths.
5. Wear reflective stripes at night.
6. Wear bright colors.
7. Choose familiar areas.
8. Walk with a companion.
9. Don't wear jewelry. Carry a whistle or mace.
10. Avoid dark isolated areas.

Walking Guidelines for Seniors

Walking is a great exercise for any age. Even in the ninth and tenth decades of life walking can improve strength and function, delay disability and improve longevity. A recent study published in *The New England Journal of Medicine* (1998) has shown that "regular walking is associated with a lower overall mortality rate in older physically capable men." For enjoyable and safe walking, here are ten guidelines for seniors:

1. Walk in optimum environmental conditions. Avoid rain, snow and heavy winds.
2. Start slow and increase pace gradually. Spend ten minutes cooling down.
3. Increase distance and decrease pace as you get older. Condition yourself.
4. Wear proper clothes, sunglasses, gloves, hats and good shoes.
5. Avoid uneven walkways to prevent falls.
6. Avoid walking in the dark.
7. Go with a spouse or friend.
8. Walk in areas familiar to you or close to your home.
9. Walk within the limits of your body—stop if you get short of breath or feel chest pain or if you become tired. Ask your physician for additional guidelines.
10. Remain alert.

References

Effects of walking on mortality among non-smoking retired men. (1998). *New England Journal of Medicine, 338*, 94-99.

Malkin, M. (1995). *Aerobic Walking.* New York, NY: John Wiley and Sons, Inc.

Meyers, C. (1992). *Walking: A Complete Guide to the Complete Exercise.* New York, NY: Random House.

Stutman, F.A. with Africano, L. (1980). *The Doctor's Walking Book.* New York, NY: Ballantine Books.

Chapter 14

Running, Safely

Walk, Don't Run

Walking is the best of all exercises. However, running is just as good for those who can do it. It is important to be fit for running. If not, running can cause problems. Here is a list of ten observed medical problems associated with jogging.

1. Muscle injuries — muscle spasms, pulled hamstrings, shin splints (injuries to muscles in front of legs), skin blisters.
2. Low back injuries, slipped disc.
3. Tendon injuries — swollen Achilles' tendon, Plantar fasciitis.
4. Bone and joint injuries — runner's knee (inflammation of the cartilage), heel spurs, stress fractures of the feet.
5. Increased incidence of osteoarthritis.
6. Sudden death (James Fixx, the author of the best-selling book *Running*, dropped dead while jogging at the age of 51).
7. Jogging induced asthma.
8. Menstrual irregularities.
9. Heat exhaustion and heat stroke.
10. Hematuria (blood in the urine) due to muscle damage.

Remember, walking briskly for one hour, five times a week, can give the same metabolic benefits as running without these risks. If you are young and fit with no musculoskeletal disabilities or any other significant medical problems, jogging is for you. It has definite advantages. You don't need special training, you can do it anywhere, it helps you burn more calories than any other aerobic exercise and it is an excellent endurance developer. But be careful when you start if you are not a regular runner.

Ten tips for novice runners:

1. Make a decision to run regularly.
2. Set aside a fixed time to run.
3. Set reasonable goals.
4. Start slow, increase speed and distance very gradually.
5. Be consistent, avoid periods of inaction. Don't look for excuses.
6. Get a thorough medical checkup before starting.
7. Make running a priority.
8. Run with a companion.
9. Be thoroughly familiar with warm-up and stretching exercises.
10. Use shoes with hard sole and soft cushioning.

Right ways to run

As with everything you do in life, there is a right way and a wrong way to do things. We discussed ten right ways to walk. Now, let us list the ten right ways to run:

1. Select the right time to run; avoid adverse weather.
2. Don't forget to warm-up and cool down.
3. Run within the limits of your fitness. Don't run too fast.
4. Maintain an erect posture.
5. Adopt a soft touch.
6. Don't run on the balls of your feet.
7. Don't overstride or understride.
8. Focus on moving forward.
9. Vary pace.
10. Relax and breathe.

Chapter 15

Bicycling for One Hundred Years

"Death may have no motion, but the bicycle is, most emphatically not its slave."

– James E. Starrs, *The Noiseless Tremor*

Any mother who carries a baby in her womb knows that a human being learns to peddle before he or she ever learns to crawl or walk. That being true and since this book is about helping you to live to be 100, you have a full century of biking in your life time. Anyone can learn to ride a bike, and the bicycle is one of the most affordable forms of exercise available to you.

This chapter presents the basic principles of biking as well as the benefits and safety measures of bike riding, all in the interest of health. Most of the information provided is for the largest segment of bikers—those who use the bicycle for outings, relaxation, exercise, and social interaction. The concerns of physical limitation and medical problems are addressed especially for the benefit of senior citizens. Of course, it is also for all those who use biking for aerobic exercises designed to promote health. Let us see the art and science of bicycling for fitness, health, and longevity.

Elements of Preparation

Anyone who wants to take up bicycling for the long haul, should pay attention to the following elements of preparation:

1. Evaluation of personal fitness.
2. Training.
3. Stretching Techniques.
4. Bicycle.
5. Helmet, shoes, clothing.
6. Nutrition, hydration.
7. Safety factors.
8. Basic principles.
9. Benefits and risks of bicycling.
10. Goals.

1. Let Your Doctor Assess Your Fitness to Bicycle

Children usually have no physical problems riding a bike. Young adults who undertake serious tasks of long distance biking, slope riding or mountain climbing are usually well informed and trained. The older population, on the other hand, may have health handicaps such as arthritis, heart disease, diabetes, stomach or urinary problems, as well as problems of poor vision or hearing. For some, obesity is also a problem. It is important to visit your physician to get a complete evaluation of your medical problems and receive clearance before beginning to ride. Make sure that your physician specifies any limitations that you may have.

2. Training

For those who don't have adequate experience in biking, it is advisable to go through a training program. Training programs are useful in helping you to get on the bike. Your trainer will discuss several important, pertinent aspects of cycling with you.

3. Stretching Techniques

Warm-up and cool-down stretching exercises are an important prerequisite to more vigorous aerobic exercises. They stimulate the mind, loosen the joints, and relax the muscles. The whole body gets ready for more activity. Stretching exercises may be done in the house or started on the street before you get on the bike. (Stretching exercises are fully discussed in Chapter 13 for your reference.) A leisurely, slow-paced ride for 5–10 minutes can serve the purpose of warm-up stretching. After the bicycling session another slow ride for 5–10 minutes can serve as a cool-down.

4. Bicycle

When selecting a bicycle, you should consider how you plan to use the bicycle. A good bicycle shopkeeper can advise you on the appropriate selection for you. A bicycle purchased for leisure riding and aerobic exercises on local streets should be comfortable and of the correct height. It should have a saddle suitable to you and gears that can be changed effortlessly. It should be fitted with reflectors in the front and back.

5. Helmet, Shoes, Clothing

You must always wear a helmet when you are riding a bike. Therefore, the helmet should be bought when you buy the bicycle. The helmet will prevent serious injuries to the head and neck. One of the biggest risks is being hit by a car. Even in areas where there are no cars, there might be several other bicycles on the bike path. Collisions can occur with skates, high speed bikes and inexperienced riders. If you are riding in a relatively risky area use knee, shin and elbow pads (McCallum, 1993). The shoes should fit comfortably and the laces should be securely tied to prevent them from being caught in the chain. The clothes should be selected on the basis of weather.

6. Nutrition, Hydration

Eating right before and after bicycling is important. Proper eating plays a large part in increasing your performance. Eat nutritious meals on the days before long distance bicycling. Eat a breakfast with fruit, whole grain cereal, and bread. During the ride take a break and eat before you feel hungry. Items such as cookies, dates, and bananas are filling and easy to carry. Do not start riding right after a heavy meal.

Staying hydrated while bicycling is also important. The body can lose fluids as perspiration especially if the weather is warm and humid. You could lose one quart of water during one hour of moderate bicycling. You must replace the lost fluid to offset dehydration and supplement the body's carbohydrate stores. For rides under two hours, it is recommended that you drink six to twelve ounces of water every 15–30 minutes. For longer trips it is advisable to drink solutions with sugar, salt and electrolytes. You can carry water with you in a water bottle held on the bicycle handles. These carriers are available at most bicycle shops.

7. Safety Factors

Cycling is an easy, fun-filled, stress-free activity and it can be safe if proper safety precautions are taken. The following tips will make your biking experience safer:

1. Use a good bike with proper clothes, shoes, and pads and do not ride without a helmet.
2. Select areas that you know are safe—without parked cars or car and pet traffic, with good roads and proper lighting.
3. Getting training for precautions, proper bike use, performance, intensity, and endurance develop biking skills (McCullagh, 1995).
4. Understand your physical limitations and medical problems. Get evaluated by your physician.
5. Stretch and warm-up before engaging in rigorous aerobic biking. Increase biking gradually. And be sure to undergo a proper cool-down afterwards.
6. Ride in a group or with a companion. For recreational biking, ride with children, family or friends.
7. Obey traffic rules and laws and follow the principles described below.

8. Carry a first aid kit with antibiotic cream, band aids, elastic bandages, steri-strips, and gauze. Also carry a water bottle, tire pump and a light.
9. Be educated about nutrition and hydration.
10. Ride defensively: Be alert, see, hear and be seen (Deburg, 1974). Use rear view mirrors, head lights, tail lights.

8. Basic Bicycling Principles

1. Obey laws, rules, traffic lights, stop signs, and school signs.
2. Ride on the right side of the street or road.
3. Yield to cars, crossing traffic of children, walkers, and joggers.
4. Yield to traffic if you are changing lanes.
5. Keep proper positions at intersections and turns.
6. Have reflectors on your bike or clothing.
7. Signal your intentions clearly when changing lanes or turning.
8. Render help if you see an injured or sick person.
9. Do not wear head phones while bicycling.
10. Do not go biking if you are sick.

9. Benefits and Risks of Bicycling.

Biking can be very safe. Only when the general biking principles and the safety tips are not followed do accidents occur. Usually the injuries are minor unless a moving automobile hits the cyclist. Nevertheless, biking is a very beneficial activity. It is a great health giver in several ways (Krausz and Krausz, 1982):

1. Bicycling is a relaxing exercise and a great way to relieve stress.
2. It is therapeutic for people with arthritis of the hips, knees and ankles. Sports medicine experts recommend bicycling for joint problems.
3. It helps you burn calories and lose weight.
4. It improves the respiratory system by increasing your respiratory capacity.
5. It improves the circulatory system by making it more dynamic. It improves cardiac output and contractility of the heart. Cardiologists use it for cardiac rehabilitation.

6. It improves appetite and digestion.
7. Elimination of waste is made faster by bicycling.
8. Muscles of the lower extremities become stronger with better tone.
9. Bicycling improves sleep.
10. Bicycling improves general health and fitness and promotes longevity.

10. Bicycling for Exercise: Goals

In one of the best books on the subject, *Fitness Cycling*, Carmichael and Burke, present in a simple way various levels of exercise. For general health and fitness, they recommend riding 20 to 60 miles, three to five days per week. Since our goal for this chapter is to present the benefits of biking that enhance health and fitness, only the details of low intensity biking are discussed. For optimum results go through the following steps:

1. Stretch or walk before bike warm-up.
2. Bike warm-up: Start biking and slowly increase your speed for 5-10 minutes to raise the heart rate to about 100 beats per minute.
3. Total 30 minute steady bike ride: Warm-up for five minutes, ride the bike for a distance of five miles in 20 minutes. Cool-down for five minutes. You will burn 31 calories per mile.
4. Total 40 minute steady bike ride: Warm-up for five minutes. Ride eight miles in 30 minutes. Cool-down in five minutes. You will burn 31 calories per mile.
5. Total 40 minute steady ride on stationary bike: Warm-up for five minutes, bike for 30 minutes, cool-down for five minutes. You will burn 7–8 calories per minute.
6. Total 55 minute variable intensity bike ride: Warm-up five minutes, bike for 12 miles in 45 minutes, cool-down for five minutes. You will burn 31 calories per mile.
7. Bike cool-down: After you complete exercise biking, lower cycling speed by using lower gear and ride for five minutes to bring the heart rate down to 120 beats per minute.
8. Enjoy bicycling, vary your route to take in new scenery; invite a riding partner.

9. Be safe while riding—avoid unknown routes or damaged roads, wear your safety gear.
10. Now you have all the basic information about bicycling. Use it wisely and safely to build better health and live longer. Take the prescription from Fausto Coppi: "Ride a bike, ride a bike, ride a bike."

References

Deburg, F. (1974). *Deburg's Guide to Bicycles and Bicycling.* Radnor, PA: Chilton Book Company.

Krausz, J. and Krausz V.V. (1982). *The Bicycling Book.* New York, NY: The Dial Press.

McCallum, P. (1993). *Spinning, A Complete Guide to the World Cycling.* Cincinnati, OH: Betterway Books.

McCullagh, J.C. (1995). *Cycling for Health, Fitness and Well-Being.* New York, NY: Dell Publishing.

Chapter 16

❦ ❦

Water Exercises

Water is a user-friendly, motivating, and enjoyable environment for exercises. Water stretching exercises and aqua aerobic exercises are easy, safe, and very effective for mental and physical relaxation, muscle strengthening, toning, weight control and total body fitness. Water exercises are good for all ages. Exercises in water allow involvement of all parts of the body. They are stimulating, and invigorating. They are good for health and longevity. Here is a simple summary of the general and medical benefits of water exercises; and all you need to know about stretching exercises, aqua aerobics and safety tips.

Ten General Benefits of Water Exercises

The following give an overview of the general benefits of water exercises. For more detailed information the reader is referred to a book by Martha White (1995):

1. Increased strength and stamina. Water exercises make you move all the time and you put in more effort than you realize. You work against the water's resistance. This results in increased expenditure of energy and the outcome is better strength and stamina.
2. Improved range of motion and better skills in moving. Due to reduced stress on muscles, joints and bones, you move better with greater range. This is especially good for people with joint disabilities.

3. Increased flexibility. Aging tends to slow down the muscle and joint capabilities. They become stiff. Water exercises loosen up the musculoskeletal system and improve flexibility.
4. Increased agility both mentally and physically. This occurs because overall water creates alertness and relaxes muscles and joints.
5. Improved balance and coordination.
6. Improved sense of well being and safety. This results in improved ability to cope with stress, improved energy level, and self-image.
7. Improved posture and appearance.
8. Increased functional strength and restoration of pain-free function. Water exercise creates improved capacity for work, better sleep, less fatigue, and more relaxation.
9. Increased aerobic endurance.
10. Greater availability. Personal swimming pools, pools in hotels while you are on a vacation or business trip, pools in gymnasiums and other places make it convenient to do water exercises. Some places offer group training sessions and some have Jacuzzis.

Ten Medical Benefits of Water Exercises

Water is therapeutic and can cause several physical and physiological changes resulting in alleviation of some medical problems (Huey and Forster, 1993). Ten significant benefits are listed below:

1. Improved circulation with improved blood supply to muscles and heart.
2. Improved oxygen consumption.
3. Greater calorie expenditure. The energy utilizing system has to work harder in water than in air. A one-hour walking workout in water burns about 500 calories compared to about 250 calories burned while walking slow on land.
4. Lowered blood pressure.
5. Reduced stress.
6. Better sleep.

Water Exercises 173

7. Improved muscle tone, increased functional strength and restoration of pain-free function.
8. Improved cardiac output.
9. Improved body composition. Water aerobic exercises are good fat burners, reducing weight and the risk of heart disease (Gaines, 1993).
10. Increased aerobic endurance. Effortless exercises improve arthritic conditions.

Ten Preparatory Guidelines

It is important to prepare yourself for water exercises before you start. This will help you enjoy the exercises, maximize your health benefits, reduce your risk of injuries and assure safety. The following ten guidelines sum up the preparations for water exercises:

1. Wear comfortable bathing clothes that are form fitting but not tight and do not slip or slide up and down.
2. Avoid eating 1 1/2 to 2 hours before water workouts. Make sure someone is around. Do not drink alcohol before a water workout.
3. Make sure the water temperature and humidity are right. Work out in the proper depth of water.
4. Take even, deep breaths at all times.
5. Avoid hyperextension of joints and maintain balance.
6. Begin exercises slowly. Increase workouts gradually. Do not overdo it to a point of tiredness, shortness of breath, or dizziness.
7. Exercise all body parts evenly.
8. Avoid range of movements beyond the normal range and comfort level.
9. Get the aerobic intensity to a level where you breathe somewhat heavily but can still talk while exercising. When you feel a sense of difficulty or pain, slow down or stop. Work out within the limits of the heart and the lungs. Take steps to prevent blisters on your feet by wearing special underwater slippers.
10. If you have any medical problems such as heart disease, breathing problems, injuries, infections, or hydrophobia (fear of water) consult your physician before you start water exercises.

Ten Stretching Exercises in Water

Now, let us present the steps of stretching and water exercises. Since this is a book for all ages, the exercises are chosen carefully to accommodate the need of persons young and old. They are thoughtfully chosen so that they will be safe for everyone. In this section the stretching exercises are presented first, to prepare you for the follow up workouts in water.

Exercise One: Water Walk

1. Stand in chest-deep water with abdominal muscles firm, tailbone pointed to floor, chest in neutral position and shoulders slightly backward. Walk slowly (Diagram 14).
2. Take deep breaths in and exhale a few times.
3. Walk forward and backwards a few times, maintaining a neutral position.
4. Push your arms forward and backwards on the side of the body as you walk.
5. Let the upper extremities move in the opposite direction of your legs while walking, i.e., your right arm should move forward as your left leg moves backwards.
6. Increase walking by taking longer steps.
7. Walk in a circle for variation.
8. Take faster steps.
9. Walk for about three minutes.
10. Stop and take a few deep breaths in and exhale.

Exercise Two: Swirling Arms

1. Stand in shoulder-deep water.
2. Extend your arms fully sideways.
3. Stand erect with your feet about 12 inches apart.
4. Rotate arms forward in small circles a few times.
5. Rotate arms backward in small circles a few times (Diagram 15).
6. Increase the circumference of circular movements and do forward circles a few times.

7. Do backward circles a few times with an increased circle circumference.
8. Do arm circles somewhat faster for variation.
9. Do this routine for three minutes.
10. Stop, breathe in and exhale a few times.

Exercise Three: Arms Water Push

1. Stand in chest-deep water.
2. Stand erect with your feet six inches apart. Extend your arms fully side ways to bring them parallel to the water's surface.
3. With your palms towards the bottom of the pool, push your arms down to your hips without bending at the elbows (Diagram 16).
4. Then reverse the position of your arms by swinging them back to the sides parallel to the surface of the water.
5. Keep your fingers close together when moving your arms.
6. Increase the speed of moving the arms up and down somewhat.
7. For variation, use hand paddles.
8. Repeat the above routine in chin deep water.
9. Spend about five minutes for this exercise.
10. Don't forget breathing in and out a few times.

Exercise Four: Side Swings

1. Stand in waist-deep water.
2. Keep your feet shoulder-width apart.
3. Extend your arms fully above your head with your palms forward.
4. Sway the arms to one side of the body enough to feel a stretch in the ribs and chest muscles (Diagram 17).
5. Sway the arms in the opposite direction.
6. Do the to-and-fro swaying on both sides a few times.
7. With hands together and the arms fully extended sway the upper extremities in a circle a few times in front of the chest.
8. Repeat the exercises slightly faster.
9. Spend about three minutes for this exercise.
10. Breathe deeply and exhale a few times.

Exercise Five: Leg Stretches

1. Stand in chest-deep water with your back resting against the pool wall.
2. With your left leg straight, flex the right hip and knee to bring the knee upward.
3. Release and straighten the right knee to let the foot go down to the floor of the pool.
4. Extend the whole right lower extremity forwards if possible to a 90-degree angle (Diagram 18).
5. Bring the right extremity down to rest the right foot on the floor.
6. Repeat the same with the right leg straight and the left lower extremity performing the same movements, as did the right.
7. Alternate the right and left leg movements a few times.
8. Repeat the exercise a few times with increased speed.
9. Carry out this activity for about three minutes.
10. Breathe deeply and exhale, a few times.

Exercise Six: Backward Leg Stretch

1. Stand in chest-deep water.
2. Hold the pool wall with left hand.
3. Stand on left foot.
4. Bend right leg backward.
5. Try to bring the heel of the right foot as close to the right buttock as possible grasping the ankle with right hand (Diagram 19).
6. Stand in this position for a few moments.
7. Bring the right foot down to rest on the floor of the pool.
8. Repeat the same on left side, facing the opposite side and holding the pool wall with right hand.
9. Perform this movement for three minutes.
10. Take a few deep breaths in and exhale fully each time.

Exercise Seven: Calf Stretch

1. Stand in chest-deep water.
2. Face the side of the pool and hold the edge of the side wall with two hands.

3. Bring left leg forward, bend the knee to bring it directly above the heel.
4. Take the right leg backwards in a straight position (Diagram 20).
5. Let the right heel press down on the floor.
6. Make sure one foot is in front of the other.
7. Relax the calf muscles to prevent an uncomfortable feeling.
8. Repeat the procedure with the other side.
9. Spend three minutes doing this.
10. Breathe in and exhale right after the procedure.

Exercise Eight: Back Stretch

1. Stand in chest-deep water.
2. Stand straight facing the side of the pool and hold onto the deck with two hands.
3. Keep the body in an arched push up position standing on the balls of the feet.
4. Then put your feet flat on the floor; push hips and the body backward.
5. Bring the body in a completely arched position.
6. Hold onto the deck, keep the body in the arched position for a few moments (Diagram 21).
7. Gradually bring the hips, body and the head out of the arched position.
8. Turn the arched position into a rounded position by straightening the elbows.
9. Repeat the exercise for about three minutes.
10. Do breathing exercises.

Exercise Nine: Body Stretch

1. Stand in shoulder-deep water.
2. Face the side of the pool and hold onto the deck with two hands.
3. Bend the knees and place toes against the wall about two feet below the hands (Diagram 22).
4. Then extend the elbows and knees to make the legs straight.
5. Maintain the position for a few moments.

6. Slowly return to the standing position.
7. Repeat the procedure a few times.
8. For variation perform the same procedure with the feet slightly apart.
9. Spend about three minutes doing this.
10. Breathe in and out.

Exercise Ten: Balancing Stretches

1. Stand in chest-deep water.
2. Stand erect and swing left arm and right leg forward.
3. Repeat the above procedure on the opposite side.
4. Stand erect and swing right leg out to the right and both arms to the left.
5. Repeat the above procedure the same way on the opposite side.
6. Stand erect and swing the right arm forward flexed at the elbow and right leg backwards flexed at the knee (Diagram 23).
7. Repeat the above procedure on the left side.
8. Repeat all of the above procedures sequentially.
9. Spend about three minutes stretching the front, side and back
10. Do breathing exercises.

Ten Aerobic Exercises in Water

Once you complete the stretching exercises, your body is ready to handle more vigorous aerobic water exercises. If your physical condition permits you to go beyond the stretching maneuvers, then undertake the following simple aerobic steps. Again, ten exercises are selected with safety as a major consideration, especially for senior citizens. Perform the exercises within the limits of your personal physical endurance. Duration of exercise is mentioned for general guidance only. For more vigorous water enthusiasts, additional aerobic exercises can be found in the books by Katz (1985), Kelly (1993) and Krasevec and Grimes (1996).

Water Exercises

Exercise One: Cardiovascular Workout Walk

1. Stand erect in neck-deep water.
2. Walk forwards, backwards and sideways as follows.
3. Swing right arm forward and left leg backwards as you walk forwards.
4. Then swing left arm forward and right leg backwards as you walk forward.
5. Repeat steps 3 and 4 as you walk forwards.
6. Reverse the movements and repeat steps 3 and 4 as you walk backwards.
7. Swing right leg to your right side and follow with the left leg as you walk to your right.
8. Swing left leg to your left side, follow with the right leg as you walk to your left (Diagram 24).
9. Exercise for three minutes.
10. Do breathing exercises.

Exercise Two: Aqua jog

1. Stand in chest-deep water.
2. Run in place.
3. Lift knees as high as possible.
4. For variation run forwards and backwards.
5. Flex elbow up to 90-degree angle as you jog.
6. Swing arms in alternating forward position (Diagram 25).
7. Relax and perform the exercise in shallow water.
8. For more energy expenditure, run in deep water again.
9. Run for three minutes.
10. Breathe in deep and exhale, a few times.

Exercise Three: Side jumps

1. Stand erect in shoulder-deep water.
2. Press feet down until your legs are straight.
3. Jump and separate legs as far as comfortably possible.

4. Keep arms stretched horizontally at start.
5. Swing arms down to touch hips coordinating with leg movements.
6. Bring your legs together and take your arms to the horizontal position (Diagram 26).
7. As you do above, squeeze the muscles of your abdomen and buttocks.
8. For variation, bend your knees slightly and repeat above exercises.
9. Exercise for three minutes.
10. Do breathing exercise with deep inhalations and exhalations.

Exercise Four: Aqua Jump

1. Stand erect in shoulder-deep water with your back against the wall.
2. Put your feet together with the soles firmly in contact with the floor.
3. As you jump, separate the legs to bring them in to an inverted "V" position.
4. Keep your arms in a horizontal position at the start.
5. As you jump and separate the legs, swing the arms straight above your head to make palms meet (Diagram 27).
6. Bring the legs together and as you do that, bring the arms back to a horizontal position.
7. For variation, as you bring the legs together swing the arms down to the sides of the hips.
8. Exercise for three minutes.
9. Breathe in deep and exhale. Do this a few times.

Exercise Five: Bike Peddling

1. Stand in chest-deep water at the corner of the pool with your back against the wall.
2. Hold onto the edge of the pool with your arms extended sideways.

3. Keep your feet firmly in contact with the floor at the start.
4. Move your legs as if you are peddling a bike (Diagram 28).
5. Do paddling for a minute.
6. Reverse paddling movement.
7. Paddle for a minute.
8. Return to paddling movement as in Step 4.
9. Exercise for three minutes.
10. Relax and do breathing exercises.

Exercise Six: Side Swiping

1. Stand in chest-deep water with your back against the wall at the corner of the pool.
2. Keep both feet firmly in contact with the floor.
3. Keep your left leg straight and bring your right leg to the side.
4. Swing your right leg downward and then across the standing left leg in a semicircular pattern (Diagram 29).
5. Bring both legs in standing position.
6. Repeat the exercise with the right leg straight and the left leg to the side and then across the right leg.
7. For variation, swing the leg in a smaller circle with the other knee slightly bent.
8. For a greater challenge, do the exercise without holding onto the wall.
9. Workout for three minutes.
10. Breathe in and out.

Exercise Seven: Leg Swinging

1. Stand in chest-deep water with back against the wall in the corner of the pool.
2. Hold onto the edge of the pool with arms on sides.
3. Flex arms slightly at elbows.
4. Keep feet firmly on floor of the pool.
5. Lift both legs together and straight and swing them to the right.
6. Keep legs together and swing them to the left (Diagram 30).

7. For variation bend the knees slightly as you swing the legs to and fro.
 8. For extra challenge extend the arms and repeat the exercise.
 9. Do the exercise for three minutes.
10. End with breathing exercises.

Exercise Eight: Leg Circling

 1. Stand in chest-deep water.
 2. Keep feet firmly on floor of the pool.
 3. Lift right leg and extend it as far as it can be done comfortably with the left leg straight.
 4. Move the right leg in a circular movement under water clockwise.
 5. Move right leg in a circular movement under water counter-clockwise.
 6. Bring the right leg in straight standing position and extend the left leg forwards.
 7. Move the left leg in a circular movement under water clockwise (Diagram 31).
 8. Move the left leg in a circular movement under water counter-clockwise.
 9. Exercise for three minutes.
10. End with breathing routine.

Exercise Nine: Body Rotating

 1. Stand erect in neck-deep water.
 2. Keep feet firmly on floor of the pool.
 3. Keep legs straight.
 4. Flex arms about 90-degrees at elbows.
 5. Rotate the torso and shoulders to the left (Diagram 32).
 6. Rotate the torso and shoulders to the right.
 7. For variation do the same with knees slightly flexed.
 8. For added difficulty hold light weights in hands.
 9. Do this for three minutes.
10. Breathe right.

Water Exercises

Exercise Ten: Combination Exercising

1. Stand erect in shoulder-deep water.
2. Keep legs straight and feet firmly on floor of the pool and criss-cross arms in front of your chest forwards and backwards with palms facing forwards and backwards, respectively (Diagram 33).
3. Flex and extend neck a few times.
4. Rotate head a few times.
5. Rotate the shoulders in an up and down circular rotation movement.
6. Stretch arms in front, palms down and fingers open. Move the arms up and down under water.
7. Bend the torso to the right and to the left a few times.
8. Jump up and down flexing the knees alternately.
9. Enjoy the combination for three minutes.
10. Relax and enjoy fresh air. Breathe in deep and exhale.

Summary

There is no better place than water to exercise, lose weight, tone up, feel free, relax, be healthy, and live longer.

Our prescription: Be a water bug.

Diagram 14

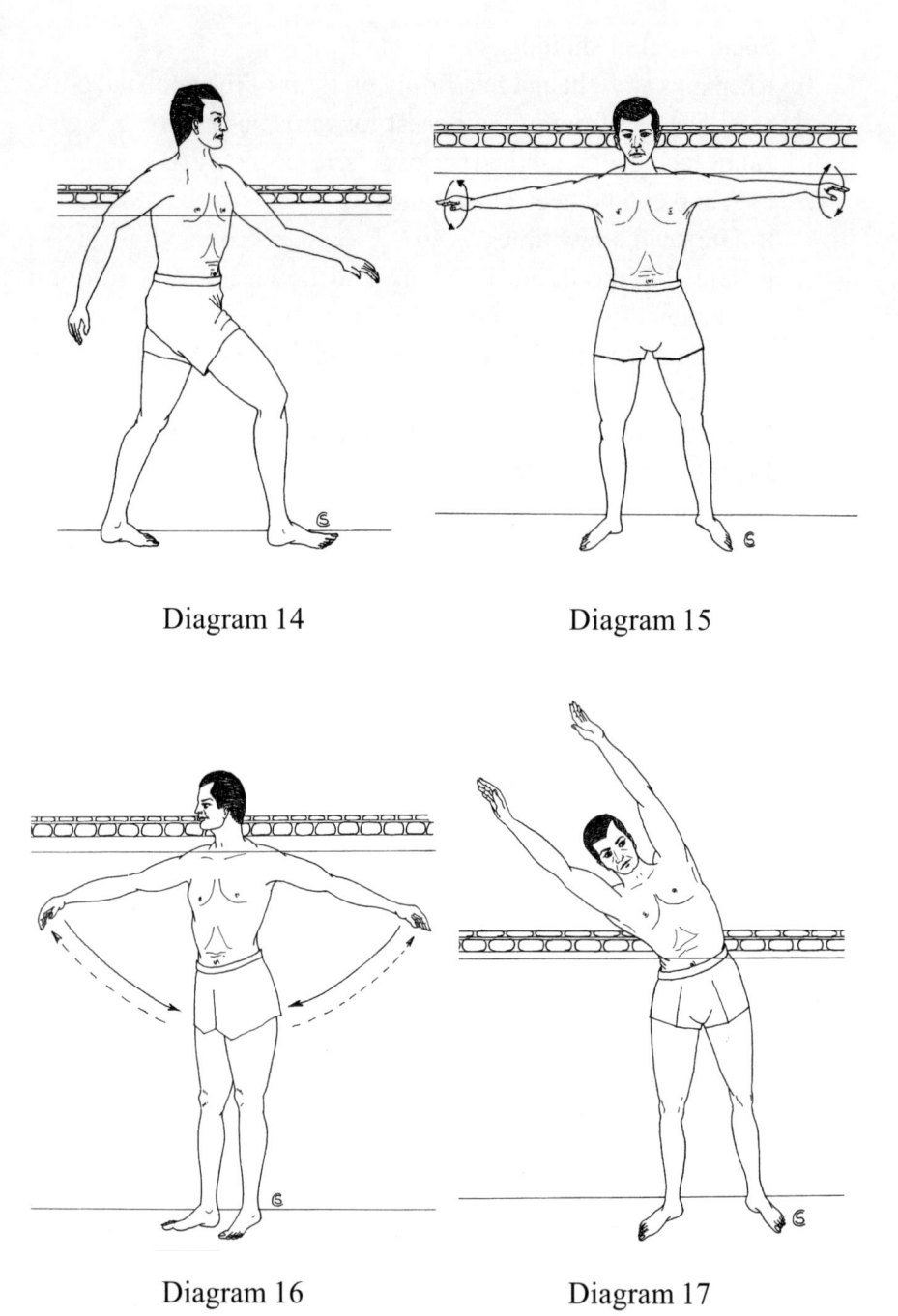

Diagram 15

Diagram 16

Diagram 17

Water Exercises

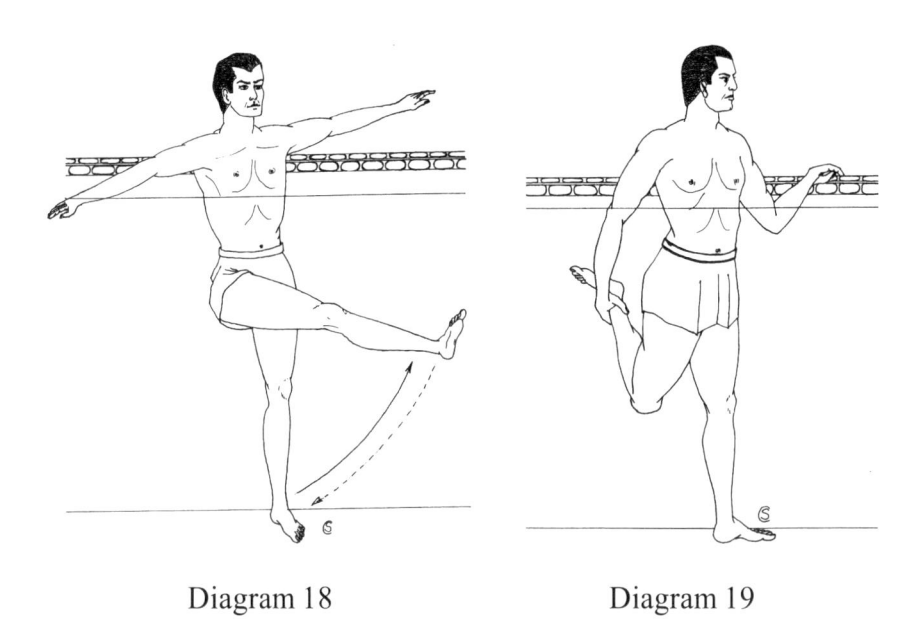

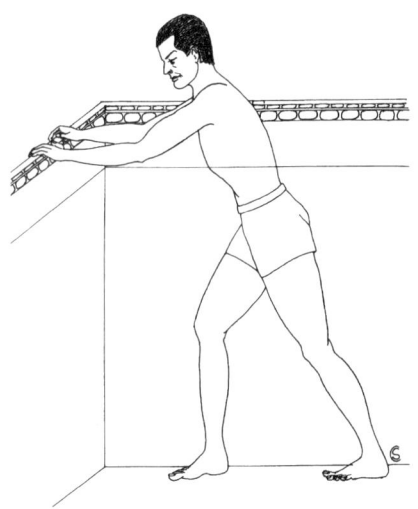

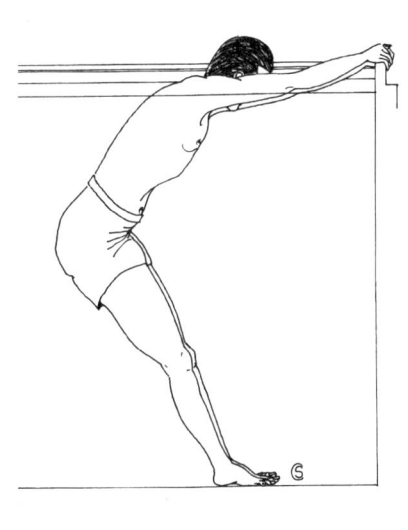

Diagram 18

Diagram 19

Diagram 20

Diagram 21

Diagram 22

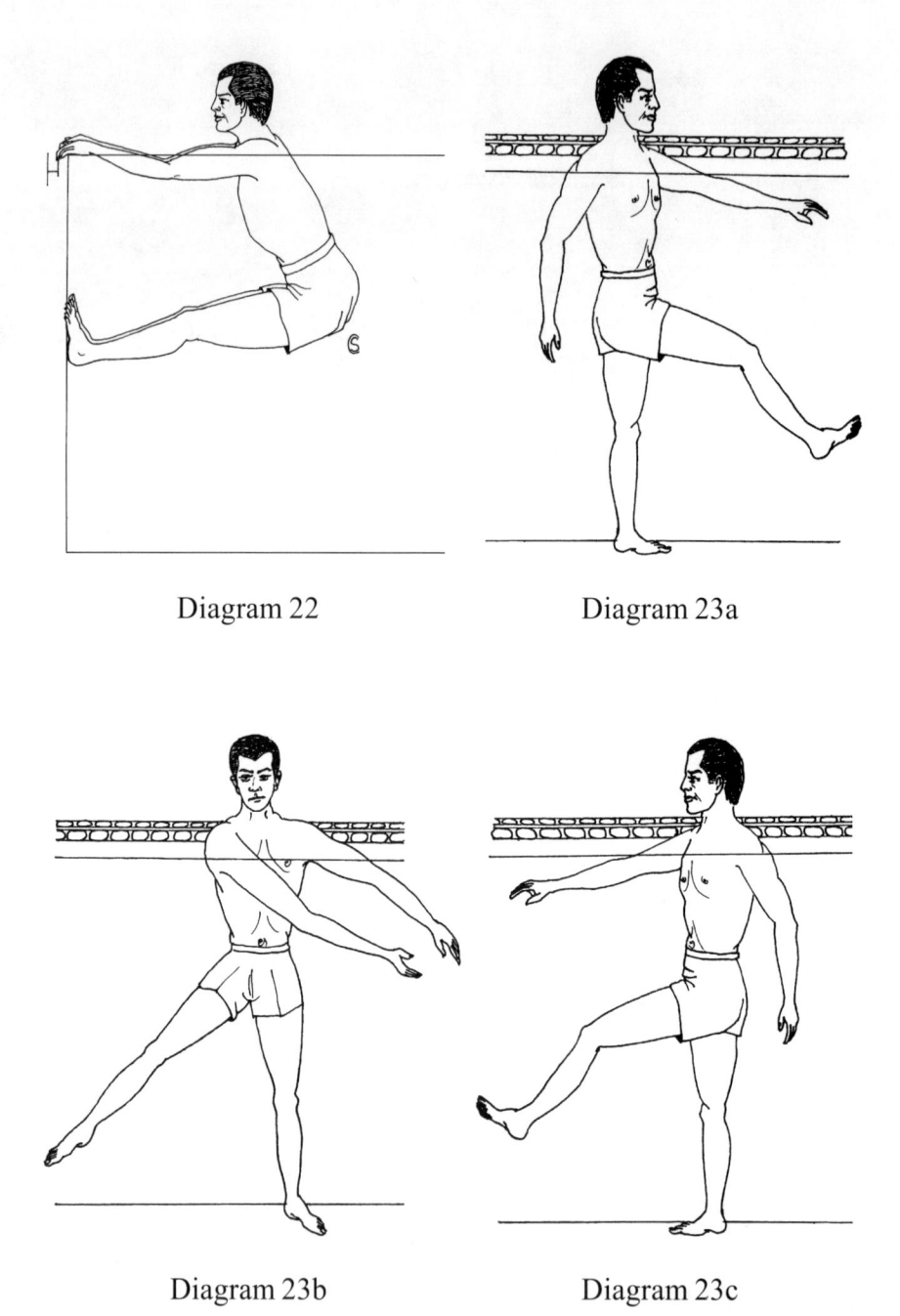

Diagram 23a

Diagram 23b

Diagram 23c

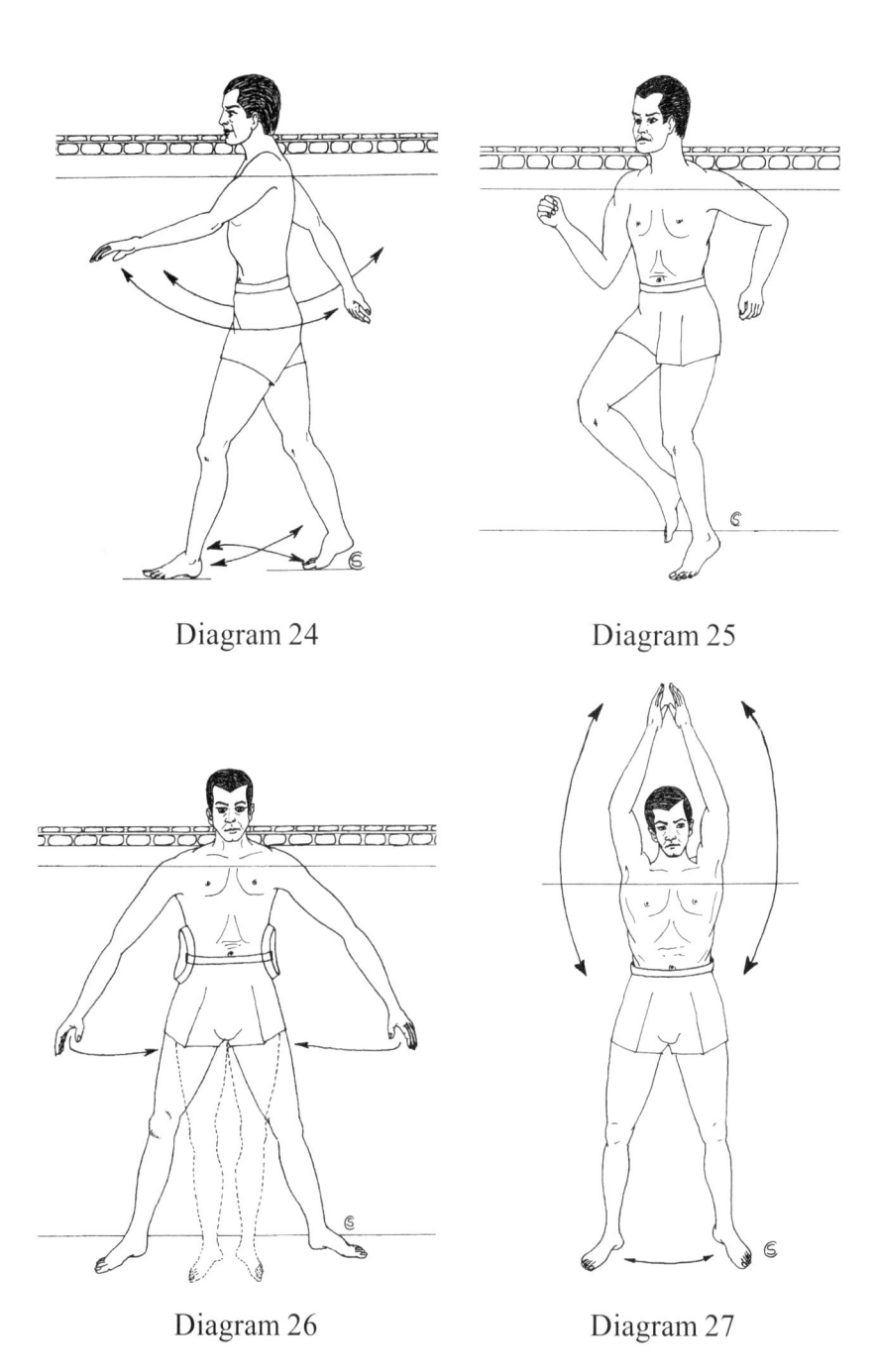

Water Exercises

Diagram 24

Diagram 25

Diagram 26

Diagram 27

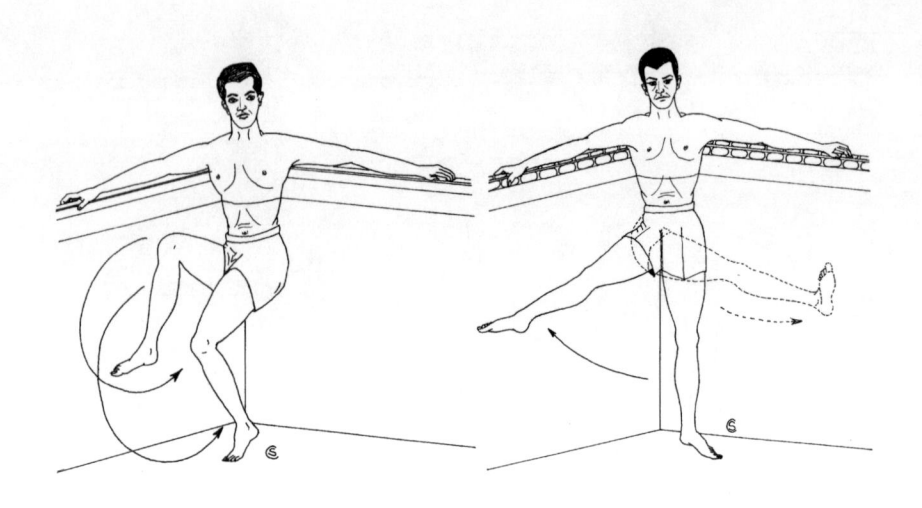

Diagram 28

Diagram 29

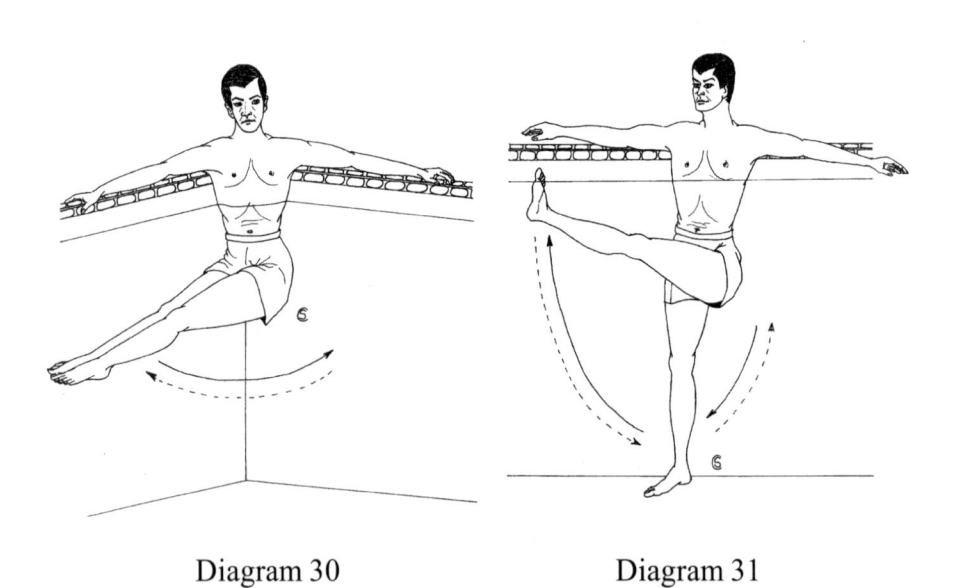

Diagram 30

Diagram 31

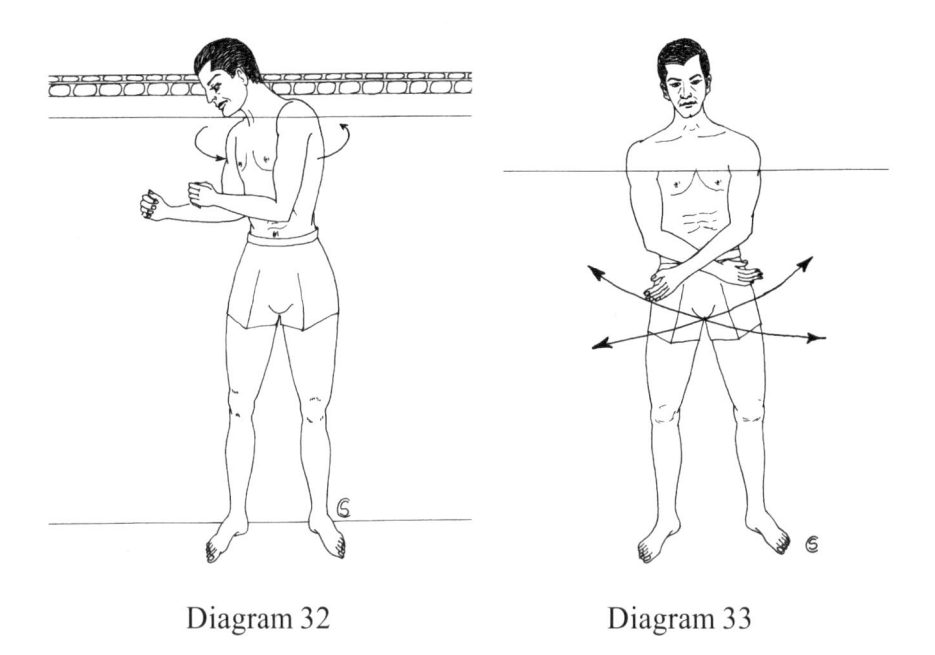

Water Exercises 189

Diagram 32

Diagram 33

References

Forster, R. and Huey, L. (1993). *The Complete Water Power Workout Book*. New York, N.Y.: Random House Publishers.

Gaines, M.P. (1993). *Fantastic Water Workouts*. Champaign, IL: Human Kinetics Publishers.

Grimes, D.C. and Krasevec, J.A. (1996). *HydroRobics*. Champaign, IL: Leisure Press.

Katz, J. (1985). *The W.E.T. Workout*. New York, NY: Facts on File Publications.

Kelly, D.V. (1993). *Aquaaerobics, Sr. Easy Pool Exercises for Senior Citizens*. Largo, Fl: Top of the Mountain Publishing.

White, M. (1995). *Water Exercise*. Champaign, IL: Human Kinetics Publishers.

Section V.

Life Style Changes and Longevity

Chapter 17

❧ ❧

Smoking

Wake Up Call

Ten startling facts:

1. Lung disease is the third leading cause of death in America.
2. Lung cancer is the leading cause of deaths among men and women. Up to 90% of lung cancers are caused by smoking. The American Cancer Society (ACS) estimates that in 1998 there will be about 171,500 new cases of lung cancer, 91,400 among men and 80,100 among women. Lung cancer will account for about 14% of all new cancers and about 29% of deaths from cancer. There will be an estimated 160,100 deaths from lung cancer in 1998.
3. Every year smoking kills more than 278,000 men and 152,000 women; one in five deaths in the U.S. is smoking-related (CDC May 23, 1997).
4. Each year in the U.S., second-hand smoke causes about 3,000 deaths from lung cancer in people who do not smoke.
5. About 30% of all coronary heart disease deaths in the U.S. each year are attributable to cigarette smoking (AHA, 1997).
6. The effect of living with a smoker is a 23% increase in the risk of ischemic heart disease (Law et al, 1997).
7. Smoking doubles the risk of stroke (AHA, 1997).
8. Environmental smoke is implicated in 300,000 cases and 212 deaths from pulmonary disease in young children and up to 2,700 sudden infant deaths every year (Walling, 1998).

9. Smoking is known to destroy antioxidant vitamins C and E as well as folate and vitamin B-12.
10. Smoking increases the risk of peripheral vascular disease, chronic bronchitis and emphysema.

The Centers for Disease Control (CDC, May, 1997) provided a disturbing answer to this question. Simply put cigarette smoking is the single most preventable cause of premature death. About 2.1 million Americans died from cigarette smoking from 1990 to 1994. Millions more will die prematurely if the current smoking patterns continue. The economic drain is also alarming; tobacco use cost $50 billion in 1993 in health care expenses.

If this is the toll cigarette smoking takes, why don't we do something individually and as a nation? In short, if you are a smoker, quit smoking. If you are not, discourage smoking and campaign against smoking. How do you do all this? The answers follow:

Ten Steps to Stop Smoking

We have successfully helped hundreds of patients quit smoking cigarettes. We have used several methods and believe going "cold turkey" is the best method. For the patients who could not do this we were successful with just a few sessions of hypnosis. Some did well with counseling; at times a single one-hour session produced success. Many quit smoking using a product we invented, Nic-Fit, containing Lobeline Sulfate. One of the methods that many patients chose and used successfully was Dr. Fatteh's Ten Point Slow Method to Quit Smoking.

1. Counseling session to get prepared.
2. Decide the date of action, establish the mind-set and start.
3. Get up in the morning, count the number of cigarettes you are used to smoking. Throw away the rest.
4. Smoke all of the counted cigarettes, for instance 20, no more, no less, during the whole day. Do exactly this everyday for one week.
5. Throw the smoked cigarette away every time when it is smoked halfway down its length. (This by itself reduces your smoking by 50%).

6. Starting the next week count 18 cigarettes and throw away the rest and smoke all 18 cigarettes, no more, no less, each day for a week, throwing each away at the half-way mark.
7. During the following weeks smoke two fewer cigarettes each week, exact numbers.
8. Counseling session for positive reinforcement.
9. Smoke, but blow the smoke right out of the mouth as soon as you take a puff. Do not inhale.
10. Final counseling session for reassurance, encouragement and promise to stay quit.

Quitting cigarette smoking is difficult but with your will power and professional support you can do it.

Secondhand Smoke

Smoking is voluntary but smokers cause involuntary smoking, also called passive smoking. The U.S. Environmental Protection Agency studied the information on the effects of passive smoking in 1993 (EPA, 1999). The evidence indicates that secondhand smoke poses a significant health hazard to children and adults. Here are some noteworthy facts:

1. Passive smoke causes lung cancer.
2. Passive smoke kills about 3,000 non-smokers in the U.S. every year.
3. Secondhand smoke increases the risk of bronchitis and pneumonia in infants and children.
4. Children exposed to secondhand smoke developed reduced lung function and symptoms of cough and wheezing.
5. Fluid can build up in the middle ear due to exposure of second hand smoke.
6. Asthmatic children who are exposed to secondhand smoke suffer an increased number of asthmatic attacks and with greater severity.
7. Second-hand smoke can affect your heart. A study of 10,914 persons showed that: "Both active smoking and environment tobacco exposure (passive smoking) are associated with progression of an index of atherosclerosis" (Walling, 1998).

Knowing this, if you are a responsible person smoking cigarettes and you truly care for your spouse, children and co-workers you will do the following:

1. You will do whatever it takes to quit smoking.
2. You will not smoke around your spouse and children.
3. You will make a commitment to make your house smoke-free.
4. You will not smoke in an automobile if there are passengers in it.
5. You will not smoke in a public place close to non-smokers.
6. You will not smoke at the work place.
7. You will ensure that you put your children in smoke-free schools and care giving places.
8. You will work with your employer to promote smoke cessation programs.
9. You will be considerate and help prevent involuntary smoking. If you are pregnant you will not smoke.
10. You will join the anti-tobacco, anti-smoking crusade.

Your prescription: Help others live longer.

Smokeless Tobacco: Not the Answer

When tobacco is used without producing smoke it is called smokeless tobacco. Such use is accompanied by chewing tobacco or using snuff. Here are a few facts about using these alternative methods of using tobacco (Cancer Website, 1999):

1. The use of chewing tobacco and snuff is increasing.
2. They are not safe practices.
3. They lead to nicotine addiction.
4. Chewed snuff significantly increases the risk of oral cancer.
5. Long-term snuff use causes 50–fold increase in the risk of cancer of cheek and gum.

Anti-tobacco and the Anti-smoking Crusade

In order to get results, the crusade against tobacco and cigarette smoking must be powerfully passionate and persistently pushed. After, all millions of lives are at stake. The crusade must be multi-directional and relentless. The public at large, law makers, educators and the health care professionals should join forces to mount a frontal assault on the massive problem of tobacco use.

References

American Cancer Society. (1997). Website: http://www.cancer.org.

American Heart Association. (1997). *Cigarette Smoking, Cardiovascular Disease and Stroke.* Website: http://www.amhrt.org.

Centers for Disease Control. (1997, May 23). Facts about cigarette mortality. *CDC Fact Sheets.* Website: http://www.cdc.gov.

Cigarette smoking and progression of atherosclerosis. (1998). *Journal of the American Medical Association, 279,* 119-124.

Environmental Protection Agency. (1993, July). *Secondhand Smoke.* Website: http://www.epa.gov.

Law, M.R. et al. (1997, October). Environmental tobacco smoke exposure and ischemic heart disease. *British Medical Journal, 315,* 973-80.

Smokeless tobacco and costs of tobacco. (1999, March 25). *Cancer Website*: http://www.cancer.org.

Walling, A.D. (1998, April 1). Effect of environmental tobacco smoke in nonsmokers. *American Family Physician, 57, 7,* 1659.

Chapter 18

Ten Best Ideas For Weight Control

"Obesity. I look upon it, that he who does not mind his belly will hardly mind anything else."

– Samuel Johnson

Obesity is a disease and it is a very common one. Thirty-three percent of the U.S. population is obese (Kuczmarski, et al., 1994).

What is obesity? The definition has been controversial. For years the table devised by Metropolitan Life Insurance Company has been used to define obesity. See Table 18.1 for a desired weight and matching calorie maintenance chart. Recently, Body Mass Index (BMI) has been accepted as a better way to define obesity (Kraemer, et al., 1990). BMI is calculated as follows: [weight (in kg) x height (in meters)]².

Measure your weight in pounds and height in inches and refer to the BMI Appendix A, Table 2. For adults, a healthy target is a BMI of less than 25. Now look at Table 18.2 and you will see that your health risk increases as the BMI increases. Persons with a BMI of over 25 and under 30 are considered overweight and those with a BMI over 30 are defined as obese. Table 18.2 also serves as a guide to what treatment options you should consider at different levels of the BMI.

TABLE 18.1
Desired Weight Daily Calorie Maintenance

	Women		Men	
Height	Weight (lbs)	Calories	Weight (lbs)	Calories
4'10"	90-98	1080-1170	95-105	1235-1365
4'11"	93-102	1115-1225	98-108	1275-1405
5'	95-105	1140-1260	100-111	1300-1445
5'1"	97-108	1165-1295	105-117	1365-1520
5'2"	100-111	1200-1335	110-123	1430-1560
5'3"	105-118	1250-1415	115-128	1495-1665
5'4"	110-123	1320-1475	120-133	1560-1730
5'5"	112-126	1345-1515	125-138	1625-1795
5'6"	117-130	1405-1560	130-143	1690-1860
5'7"	120-134	1440-1610	133-148	1730-1925
5'8"	125-139	1500-1670	137-153	1780-1990
5'9"	130-144	1560-1730	143-159	1860-2065
5'10"	135-149	1620-1790	148-164	1925-2130
5'11"	140-154	1680-1850	152-168	1975-2185
6'	144-158	1730-1895	155-171	2015-2225
6'1"			163-179	2120-2325
6'2"			167-183	2170-2380
6'3"			170-188	2210-2445
6'4"			172-195	2235-2535
6'5"			178-198	2315-2575
6'6"			185-206	2405-2680

Obesity is a dangerous disorder. It increases your risk of heart disease. It is associated with high blood pressure, dislipidemia, lowered HDL (good cholesterol), impaired glucose tolerance and heart failure. Look at the following ten health benefits even with a weight loss of 5-10% (Blackburn, 1995).

1. Decreased cardiovascular risk and heart failure.
2. Lower blood sugar and insulin levels and decreased risk of diabetes.
3. Decreased blood pressure.
4. Decreased LDL (bad cholesterol).
5. Decreased triglycerides.
6. Increased HDL.
7. Reduced symptoms of joint problems.
8. Improvement in gynecologic conditions.
9. Reduced sleep apnea.
10. Increased longevity (Williamson, 1997).

Obesity is a high stakes disorder economically. "It ranks among the major determinants of health care costs." (Seidell, 1995). Obesity related conditions such as diabetes, coronary heart disease, osteoarthritis, high blood pressure, gall bladder disease and some cancers cost $51.6 billion in 1995 alone. This is 5.7% of the total health expenditure in that year. The costs are due to increased numbers of office visits, increased hospitalizations, surgeries, laboratory tests and increased use of drugs.

Why are so many of us obese? Here are ten reasons:

1. Heredity plays a big part; it is blamed for 30–70% of the cases of obesity. If one parent is obese, there is a 40% chance of his or her child becoming obese. If both parents are obese, the child has a 70% chance of becoming obese.
2. High fat diet: The average American diet is too rich in fats. Forty to 50% of the calories come from fats. This is an important factor in obesity.

TABLE 18.2
BMI: Degree of Health Risk & Treatment Options

BMI	Health Risk	Treatment Option
< 25	Low	1. Sensible Eating 2. Moderate Reduction of Calories (women: 1200/ men: 1400) 3. Exercise 30 min/ 5 times/week
25 - 29	Moderate	1. Sensible Eating 2. Low Calorie Diet (women: 800-1000/ men: 1100-1200) 3. Exercise
30 - 40	High	1. Sensible Eating 2. Very Low Calorie Diet (800) 3. Exercise 4. Medication
> 40	Very High	1. Sensible Eating 2. Very Low Calorie Diet (800) 3. Exercise 4. Medication 5. Surgery

3. Reduced energy expenditure: Only 22% of the population is adequately physically active. A 54% majority are not active enough and 24% are totally sedentary (Brownell and Wadden, 1998).
4. Hypothyroidism – underactive thyroid gland.
5. Slow metabolic rate.
6. Too many fat cells (hyperplastic obesity).

7. Upbringing that promotes overeating.
8. Psychological factors: Many people overeat when they are depressed or stressed.
9. Environmental factors: Loneliness can promote overeating. Overeating also occurs at parties, buffets and all-you-can-eat places.
10. Certain medications such as oral contraceptives can cause weight gain.

We are fat. *But are we getting fatter?* Unfortunately, yes. One hundred years ago, men in their forties weighed an average of 140 pounds; now they weigh 173 pounds. Women in their forties weighed an average of 128 pounds a century ago and now they weigh an average of 140 pounds. In the past 15 years the mean weight of Americans has increased by 7.9 pounds. Americans weighed 8% less in 1985 compared to 1995.

So, what should we do? How should we do it? First, look at Table 20 to find out your desired weight and matching calorie count. Then, start with two goals: One, lose weight, and two, maintain weight. Both goals are equally important.

Managing Your Weight

Let us remember that no single drug or single approach is universally effective for losing weight. One must be prepared for a multi-faceted weight loss and maintenance effort. These are summarized in the following five steps:

Step I: Commitment and Compliance

1. Consult your physician.
2. Determine your BMI.
3. Determine the number of calories needed. Determine your calorie count.
4. Select appropriate exercises.
5. Determine treatment option.
6. Make a commitment to total compliance.

Step II: Behavior Modification

1. Remain motivated.
2. Be positive, determined and dedicated.
3. Be patient and persistent.
4. Stay busy, avoid loneliness, eat in company.
5. Reduce stress.

Step III: Exercise

1. Select the exercises suitable to you.
2. Exercise regularly.
3. Exercise five times a week.
4. Determine desired daily calorie expenditure.
5. To lose one pound a week, burn 500 calories a day. If your food gives you 1,500 calories, burn 2,000 calories by exercising. Alternatively, reduce calorie intake by 250 a day and burn 250 calories a day to achieve a loss of 500 calories.

Step IV: Sensible Eating

1. Eat a balanced nutritious low fat diet.
2. Eat at regular hours, avoid those late night binges just before going to sleep
3. Eat slowly, chew food thoroughly.
4. Avoid eating in front of the television; avoid cruises, all-you-can-eat places, and buffets.
5. Eat three meals a day: avoid snacks, soft drinks, desserts and alcohol.

Step V: Special Considerations

1. Set reasonable goals; get there slowly and gradually.
2. If you take diet pills, know the side effects and contraindications.
3. Lose weight to attain better long-term health, not just to look good for a short time.
4. After losing weight, do everything possible to maintain your new weight. Don't let a lapse cause relapse.
5. Learn to say "no" to yourself.

What about diet pills?

Many different diet pills have been used in the past. Some of them are listed in Table 18.3 (Murphy, 1999). Significant dropouts have been Redux and combinations of Phentermine and Fenfluramine called Phen-Fen because of side effects. Phentermine has been in use for many years. In his experience, Guy-Grand (1997) believes that the treatment strategies of diet, behavioral modification and exercise have been ineffective for maintaining long-term weight loss and suggests that pharmacotherapy combined with classical treatment strategies has improved the long-term maintenance of weight loss. We believe the classical strategies are effective and that pharmacotherapy does provide the incentive and contributes to better results. In our experience with hundreds of patients, of all the drugs Phentermine has been the most effective.

Xenical (Orlistat): A New Kid on the Block?

This Hoffman La Roche product, Xenical, a minimally absorbable agent, inhibits the activity of pancreatic and gastric lipases and blocks gastrointestinal absorption of dietary fat by 30%. In a study of 1,187 subjects, 60 mg or 120 mg capsules of Orlistat were given for two years together with weight maintenance, diet and behavior modification strategies. The conclusion was, "two-year treatment with Orlistat plus diet significantly promotes weight loss, lessens weight regain, and improves some obesity-related disease risk factors" (Davidson, et al, 1999).

Correction of obesity and sustained maintenance of healthy weight will significantly contribute to a decrease in the incidence of serious conditions such as heart disease, diabetes and osteoarthritis. This will result in a longer life and reduction in later-life disabilities. Here are ten best ideas for weight control:

1. Determine your BMI.
2. Determine the number of calories you need.
3. Determine the treatment option.
4. Set reasonable goals.
5. Be totally committed and remain compliant.

TABLE 18.3
Side Effects of Popular Diet Medications

Drug	Daily Dose	Side Effects
Dexatrim, Acutrim (OTC)	75 mg	Nervousness, tremor, palpitation
Biphetamine (Amphetamine) Schedule II	10-15 mg	Nervousness, tremor, palpitation
Preludin (Phenmetrazine) Schedule II	75 Mg	Palpitation, dizziness, insomnia, euphoria, tremor, headache
Didrex (Benz-phetamine HCL) Schedule III	24-150 mg	Abuse potential. Mental impairment during hazardous activity, CNS over-stimulation, arrythmia, hyper-tension, dry mouth, GI disturbance, impotence
Bontril (Phen-dimetra-minetarta-rate) Schedule III	105 mg	Dizziness, headache, tremor, agitation, blurred vision
Tenuate Dospan Schedule IV	75 mg	As with Didrex, plus seizures, blood dycrasia, shortness of breath
Fastin (Phen-termine HCL) Schedule IV	30 mg	As with Didrex, plus primary pulmonary hypertension, heart valvular disease
Ionamin (Phen-termine resin) Schedule IV	15-30 mg	Abuse potential, hypertension, arrythmia, CNS over-stimulation, dry mouth, GI disturbances, psychosis, impotence
Meridia	10-15 mg	Dry mouth, anorexia, insomnia, constipation, headache, nervousness, increased blood pressure, dizziness
Xenical (Orlistat)	240-360 mg	Oily spotting, flatus, fecal urgency, fatty stools, oily evacuation, increased defecation, and fecal incontinece

6. Modify your behavior, be positive.
7. Exercise regularly.
8. Eat sensibly.
9. Lose weight slowly and gradually.
10. Make maintenance of weight loss a lifetime effort.

References

Blackburn, G. (1995). Effect of degree of weight loss on health benefits. *Obes Res, 3* (Suppl), 211s-216s.

Browned, K.I.D. and Wadded, T.A. (1998). *The LEARN Program for Weight Control.* Dallas, TX: American Hearth Publishing Company.

Campbell, S.M., Flegal, K.M., Johnson, C.L., Kuczmarski, R.J. (1994). Increasing prevalence of overweight among U.S. adults: The National Health and Nutrition Examination Survey. *Journal of the American Medical Association, 272,* 205-211.

Davidson, et al. (1999, January 20). Weight control and risk factor reduction in obese subjects treated for two years with Orlistat. *Journal of the American Medical Association, Vol. 281, No. 3,* 235-242.

Guy-Grand, B. (1997). Pharmacological approaches to intervention. *International Journal of Obesity, 21,* (Suppl. 1), S22-S24.

Kraemer, H., Berkowitz, R.I., Hammer, L.D. *Methodological Difficulties in Studies of Obesity, I: Measurement Issues. Ann Behav Med.* 1990; 12:112-118.

Murphy, J.U.L., Ed. (1999). *Monthly Prescribing Reference.* New York, NY: Prescribing Reference, Inc.

Seedily, J.C.L. (1995). The impact of obesity on health status: Some implications for health care costs. *International Journal of Obesity, 19,* (suppl), S13-S16.

Williamson, D.F. (1997). International weight loss: Patterns in the general population in its association with morbidity and mortality. *International Journal of Obesity, 21,* (Suppl. 1), S14-19.

Chapter 19

✧ ✧

Stress Busting Strategies

Stress arises from a reaction to an adverse environment resulting in psychological and emotional negative feeling and often physical harm. Most organs in the body including the heart, brain, muscles, joints, liver, and the immune system are affected by stress. If stress is beyond the limits of tolerance, there is bodily malfunction, inhibition or breakdown of various systems (Barley and Torte, 1992). This affects longevity.

The United States is a pressure cooker society, in our opinion, a nine on a scale of one to ten, ten representing the highest degree of stress. The Japanese score a ten. A Japanese patient of ours indicated that he migrated to the U.S. because "there is a lot less stress here." On the other hand, patients from other countries readily admit that there is a high degree of stress in the U.S. The sources of stress may be physical or socio-cultural circumstances. Major life events can induce acute stress. Ten of the most stress inducing events are rated in Table 19.1 (Holes and Rae, 1967).

External/ Environmental Stress

Domestic Stress

Everyone goes through stress. Day-to-day stress plays an important part in our life. Let us examine the components of the "stresses of life." The most significant, yet least talked about, sources of external stress come from children, grandchildren, spouses, parents, and grandparents.

TABLE 19.1
Stress Level of Major Life Events

Rank	Life Event	Unit Value
1	Death of a Spouse	100
2	Divorce	73
3	Marital Separation	65
4	Jail Term	63
5	Death of Close Family Member	63
6	Personal Injury or Illness	53
7	Marriage	50
8	Fired from Work	47
9	Retirement	45
10	Marital Reconciliation	45

Everyone knows family causes stress. Children have to be driven to school, sporting events and other activities that strain the parents' ability to keep their schedules. Grandchildren are usually a source of happiness, but for a grandparent with health problems caring for children can be a burden and stress. And someone has to care for the parents and grandparents. Those who have to are required to be concerned about their needs and their health. This is stressful.

Stress arising out of spousal relationship comes from marital conflicts, sexual dissatisfaction, marital infidelity, and even worse, divorce. Divorce creates a tug of war for custody of children and the responsibility of caring for them alone. There are the added financial problems of collecting alimony. Beyond that, there is stress from adjusting to a new life and new relationships. However, the worst stress comes, of course, from the death of the spouse.

Are you one of those who have to face up to a combination of these responsibilities? If you are, God bless you, for these are formidable and stressful situations.

Job Stress

Another source of stress is the job. One may be forced to sacrifice the time needed to enjoy the pleasures of family life. It all starts at home. Think of the mornings when you have to get children ready for school and at the same time make sure you are at work on time. There is the stress of traveling to work and the problems of punctuality. Think of times when you receive calls at work concerning your child's problems with the babysitter, the daycare and school.

At work, the subordinates do not perform up to par; co-workers create friction and the boss puts pressure on you or is downright nasty. This is stressful. Sometimes you are under pressure because of job security, overtime obligations, and deadlines.

If you don't have to balance your check book day-to-day you are lucky. This is not the privilege most people have. Bills come everyday that must be paid or settled. Mortgage payments, car loan payments, and credit card liabilities must be addressed to avoid foreclosures, forfeitures, and bad credit. To make ends meet you have to stay on top of the work, be productive, and put up with nonsense. All this means more stress.

Positive and Negative Stress

Stress can be positive stress or negative. Writing this book we spent many hours beyond our working time. We enjoy doing this. For each chapter we set deadlines. This is a classic example of positive stress, which "at the end of the day," provides a lot of satisfaction. This type of stress is healthy. On the other hand, negative stress results from tasks that you have to perform even if you don't like them, such as meeting deadlines imposed by others. Such stress hurts health.

How Does Stress Affect Health and Longevity

Both acute and chronic stress can cause many medical problems. Acute stress can cause headaches, tiredness, anxiety, indigestion, diarrhea, palpitations, depression, nervousness, tremors, teeth grinding, and insomnia. It can also cause low back pain, chest pain, gastritis, nervous tics, feeling of suffocating pressure, irritability, panic attacks, lack of concentration, emotional upheaval, and over reaction to trivial matters.

Chronic stress can be associated with many additional medical maladies. It can disturb one's metabolism and induce diabetes (Wyngaarden and Smith, 1988). Severe emotional and psychological stress can cause baldness. The condition called spastic colon or irritable bowel syndrome, and peptic ulcers are often initiated or aggravated by stress. Overwhelming evidence exists documenting harmful effects of stress on the cardiovascular system (Wayne, 1998). Mental stress can produce increased heart rate, elevated blood pressure and greater cardiac output. These psychological changes can precipitate death. Stress also suppresses the immune function and can cause an increased risk of allergies and even cancers (Boca and Satin, 1997).

How Do We Create Stress?

Knowingly or unknowingly many of us create stress for ourselves. The following are ten ways self-induced stress is created:

1. We believe we have to be perfect.
2. We try to do everything ourselves.
3. We believe we must not fail.
4. We create unrealistic deadlines.
5. We don't know how to say "no".
6. We don't laugh.
7. We don't learn how to develop positive attitudes.
8. We don't develop intimacy with family, friends and co-workers.
9. We don't sleep enough.
10. We involve ourselves in unhealthy competition.

How To Banish Stress?

Now that we know how we create stress, how do we deal with it? Worry is a big component of stress (Halloween, 1997). It is important

Stress Busting Strategies

to banish worry. It can be done without medications. Ten ways to banish worry and stress are:

1. Seek advice from friends, family members and your doctor.
2. Have faith, pray, and let go of problems.
3. Get enough sleep.
4. Eat a balanced healthy diet.
5. Exercise regularly, don't slow down.
6. Do something you like. Search for what is good in life. Be alive and creative.
7. Love and be loved.
8. Spend time with people you like. Avoid loneliness.
9. Don't underestimate yourself. Be positive and upbeat.
10. Talk to yourself. Learn to cope. Coping successfully promotes health and enhances longevity.

Dealing with Acute Stress

To deal with acute stress combine the following ten stress busters with the above ways to wean off worry (Olinekova,1998):

1. Learn to relax, use meditation, yoga or prayers.
2. Find time to unwind and rest.
3. Get scalp and body massage.
4. Use stretching exercises to eliminate muscle spasms.
5. Avoid caffeine and alcohol.
6. Take a warm bath.
7. Enjoy the wonderful stress reliever, sex.
8. Laugh a lot.
9. Listen to soft music in a quiet place.
10. Watch a comedy program or movie.

Long Term Stress Busting Strategies

How do you really solve the problems of chronic stress? How do you deal with stress from major singular life events listed in Table 26. A careful analysis and the acceptance of the following ten guidelines will help you.

1. Look at all the stresses. Analyze and understand the causes of your stresses. Address the causes of self-induced stresses and systematically eliminate each.
2. Stay in shape mentally and physically. Sound mind and healthy body will be able to withstand stresses better and you will be stronger to seek the solutions and apply the effective measures to find answers better and secure peace.
3. Change the job if it is the cause of chronic stress with no hope of relief. If the nature of work becomes harder and harder to deal with, consider change of career. If survival is difficult working for others, consider self-employment.
4. Make compromises with the spouse and family members. Be considerate and equitable.
5. Drop the responsibilities that go beyond the level of comfort in handling them. Do not set unrealistic deadlines for yourself. Compete with yourself not with others.
6. Learn to say "no". Remember, the more work you do for your boss, the more work you will get. Don't be a workaholic. The same principle that goes for your boss applies to the family members. The more you give them the more they will demand.
7. Prepare for catastrophes. Accept death in the family, divorce, or any of the major life events with grace and courage.
8. Walk out of a job before you are burned out. Do not procrastinate. Reserve time for entertainment or rejuvenation.
9. Treat your health problems that increase your stress. Control pains of arthritis or any other conditions that render your mind and body functionless. Do not smoke or abuse alcohol and drugs that disable you mentally and physically.
10. If everything fails and you feel cornered or helpless, seek professional help.

So, here is our prescription: Take charge. Do whatever it takes to bust stress. You will be healthier and live longer.

References

Barley, J. and Torte, L. (1992). *Dr. Barley's Food Allergy and Nutrition Revolution.* New Can, CT: Kits Publishing, Inc.

Boca, K. and Satin, H. (1997). *The Road to Immunity. How To Survive and Thrive in a Toxic World.* New York, NY: Pocketbooks of Simon & Schuster.

Halloween, E.M. (1997). *Worry, Controlling It and Using It Wisely.* New York, NY: Pantheon Books.

Holes, D. and Rae, R. (1967). The social readjustment rating scale. *Journal of Psychosomatic Research, 11*, 213–218.

Olinekova, G. (1998). *Power Aging. Young at Any Age.* New York, NY: Thunder Mouth Press.

Smith H.L. and Wyngaarden, D.U.B., Eds. (1988). *Cecil Textbooks of Medicine.* Philadelphia, PA: WEB. Sanders Co.

Wayne, H.H. (1998). *Living Longer with Heart Disease.* Los Angeles, CA: Health Information Press, 68.

Chapter 20

❦ ❦

The Power Of Sleep

Sleep is the best invigorator of the body and mind. Good sleep is decidedly an overnight charging of the body and mind battery. Without this charging, peak performance of any of the systems is not possible. Lack of sleep literally disables the body and impairs the mind.

How Much Sleep Do We Need?

"For optimal daytime alertness, humans require about eight hours of sleep per 24-hour period" (Neubauer, 1999). However a 1993 poll by Louis Harris indicated that 50% of adult Americans do not get their full quota of natural sleep. About 25% have occasional sleeping problems and 10% have chronic problems. Working women are sleeping less now than before. The Economics Policy Institute in Washington, DC recently published the results of a study indicating that women who work have 161 fewer hours a year for sleep and leisure than their mothers did 20 years ago.

How much does an average person sleep? The National Center for Health Statistics offers the figures in Table 20.1 (Ford, 1994). This information indicates that sleeping patterns change with aging. For adults under 60, up to eight hours of sleep is adequate. After age 60, six hours of sleep may be enough. Elderly persons typically need

TABLE 20.1
Necessary Sleep Levels

Age	Average Hours of Sleep per Night
Newborn	16.5
6 months	14.0
6 years	11.0
12 years	9.0
15-19 years	8.5
20-29 years	7.5
30-49 years	7.0
50-59 years	6.75
60-79 years	6.5
> 80 years	6.0

less total night time sleep but require day time naps. We believe the best measure of adequacy of sleep is to base it on how you feel with the amount of sleep you do get.

Humans can endure extreme limits of wakefulness. The official record for going without any sleep was set by Randy Gardner in 1995 (The Guinness Book of World Records, 1998). He stayed awake for 264 hours and 12 minutes, then slept for 14 hours and 40 minutes!

Dangers of insomnia

Do you toss and turn in bed all night, every night? Do you keep looking at the clock every hour? Are you deprived of a normal quota of sleep each night? If you are, you have the problem of insomnia. This is a serious problem. Here is a list of ten dangerous side effects of insomnia (Amass, 1998):

1. Irritability leading to poor social interaction.
2. Impaired concentration and overall central nervous system malfunction resulting in poor work performance.
3. Anxiety, increased stress and lack of interest in the surrounding.
4. Drowsiness and sluggish thinking.
5. Impairment of immune system.
6. Lethargy, physical sluggishness and lack of energy.
7. Reduced ability to cope with problems.
8. Increased potential to fall asleep while driving.
9. Tendency to overeat and gain weight.
10. Chronic fatigue and even psychotic behavior with prolonged sleep deprivation.

Ten benefits of good sleep

You feel great when you sleep well. You are fresh, you sing, whistle and dance and do things with gusto. Good sleep, indeed, makes a big difference in the way you react to the world. Good sleep benefits you in ten ways:

1. It relaxes the brain, reduces stress and improves thinking.
2. It eliminates fatigue.
3. It lowers blood pressure.
4. It decreases heart rate.
5. It relaxes muscles.
6. It increases energy level and improves physical and mental performance.
7. You recover faster from illnesses.
8. Your immune system is strengthened.
9. You become nicer to people.
10. You are more confident.

TABLE 20.2
Caffeine Content in Beverages

Beverage (5 oz serving)	Caffeine Content (mg?)
Drip coffee	11-150
Percolated coffee	65-125
Instant coffee	10-110
Brewed de-caf coffee	2-5
Instant de-caf coffee	2
Tea bag, brewed 5 min.	20-50
Loose black tea, brewed 5 min.	20-55
Loose green tea, brewed 5 min.	15-80
Iced tea	20-35
Cocoa	40-50

Ten causes of insomnia

It is important to recognize the causes of insomnia because that will help you solve your sleeping problem. Here are ten causes:

1. Anxiety, stress, grief, worry, depression, excitement or exhilaration.
2. Alcoholism or abrupt cessation of alcohol intake after prolonged use.
3. Use of medications and caffeine. See Table 20.2 for the ten commonest sources of caffeine.
4. Medical conditions (see p. 222).
5. Long naps during the daytime.
6. Obesity, sleep apnea, allergies, asthma.

7. Abrupt discontinuation of sleeping pills.
8. Uncomfortable bed, bright bedroom, noisy environment.
9. Jet lag, shift work.
10. Aging.

Commandments For Good Sleep

1. Form good sleeping habits. Go to bed at a regular time. Get up at the same time every day.
2. Prepare the right environment to sleep. Follow ten specific steps listed below.
3. Take special steps to manage the problem of insomnia related to shift work.
4. Correct medical problems causing insomnia. These are discussed below.
5. Deal with snoring problem as described later.
6. Achieve muscle relaxation with exercises in bed.
7. Diffuse stress and emotional upsets using techniques described in chapter on stress.
8. Eat right. Do not go to bed immediately after a heavy meal. Do not go to bed hungry.
9. Get enough exercise during the evening to become pleasantly fatigued.
10. Avoid alcohol, coffee, tea, soft drinks for six to eight hours before bedtime.

More Specifically

Ten components of a no-drug, no-cost natural formula to fall asleep.

1. Make the bedroom sleep-inducing—quiet, dark, cool.
2. For peace and calm listen to soft music, turn off the television and, if possible, turn the telephone ringer off.
3. Use the biggest bed with the most comfortable mattress and pillows you can buy.

4. Take a warm bath. Use the grandma remedy—drink a glass of warm milk. Nowadays, a glass of warm skim milk. It contains a natural sleep-inducing amino acid.
5. Wear loose comfortable clothes.
6. Wind down, read, take a massage and do breathing exercises.
7. Enjoy sex—it is a natural sleep inducer.
8. Keep worry and work outside the bedroom.
9. Use self hypnosis or guided imagery (a technique to create mental images and self suggestions) to fall asleep.
10. Don't fight sleep. If you can't sleep, get out of bed, walk around, read again, stretch and do breathing exercises. Repeat this every 30 minutes if necessary.

Snoring and Sleep

Snoring can be a major factor in sleep deprivation. It can be a very annoying noise, causing the non-snoring sleep partner to lose sleep night after night. Snoring has resulted in many divorces! Take the following ten steps to reduce or eliminate snoring:

1. Lose weight.
2. Use less antihistamines and sleeping pills
3. Sleep on your side
4. Humidify the air in your bedroom
5. Stop smoking. Avoid alcohol
6. Raise the head of the bed
7. Correct allergies
8. Be considerate to others
9. Buy a snore control device
10. Get evaluated by an ear, nose and throat specialist to get medical treatment or possible surgical intervention.

Shift Work and Sleep

Many of us are unfortunate to have to work at night. In America, more people work night shifts than in any other country in the world. For those who have to earn their wages working nights, getting sufficient sleep can be a problem. They have to mold the body and mind and make adjustments to make life compatible to night shift working. To make the night like day and day like night, here are ten steps (Caldwell, 1997):

1. Avoid night shifts if at all possible, on the basis of family hardship and medical problems.
2. Negotiate with your employer to inform you of the night shift engagement several days in advance.
3. Ask for regular, not rotating shifts, and stay on one shift for an extended period without frequent rotation changes.
4. Prepare several days in advance for the shift work.
5. Educate your family members, especially children about your need to sleep.
6. To get adequate amount of sleep, budget your time, sleep at regular times.
7. As you do for night sleep, make your day sleeping environment conducive to good sleep. Pay special attention to darkening the room and eliminating noises. This may be slightly difficult since in daytime there is generally more light and more noise.
8. Adjust the time periods to eat, exercise and attend social functions in advance.
9. Avoid the use of alcohol, caffeine, and smoking for 6 to 8 hours before going to bed.
10. Follow the other steps described above. If you have a serious sleeping disorder, consult your physician.

Medical Conditions That Cause Sleeping Problems

It is important to treat medical conditions to prevent or cure sleeping problems. Here is a list of ten medical conditions that cause sleeping problems.

1. High blood pressure and coronary artery disease with angina
2. Enlargement of prostate
3. Bladder infection

4. Arthritis, anemia, overactive thyroid, and restless leg syndrome (uncomfortable crawling deep inside the leg muscles).
5. Hiatus hernia, gastroesophageal reflux causing heartburn.
6. Anxiety, stress and depression
7. Allergies, asthma, and chronic obstructive pulmonary disease.
8. Alcoholism and nicotine addiction
9. Obesity and sleep apnea
10. Headaches

Our prescription: Sleep is great medicine, get enough.

References

Neubauer, D.N. (1999, May 1). Sleep problems in the elderly. *American Family Physician, Vol. 59, No. 9*, 2551

Ford, N. (1994). *The Sleep Rex. 75 Proven Ways to Get a Good Night's Sleep.* Englewood Cliffs, N.J: Prentice Hall.

The Guinness Book of World Records. (1998). Stanford, CT: Guinness Media, Inc.

Amass, J.A.B. (1998). *Power Sleep.* New York, NY: Viler.

Caldwell, J.P. (1997). *Sleep. Everything You Need to Know.* Buffalo, NY: Firefly Books.

Chapter 21

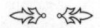

❦ ❦

Love

"I am not aware of any other factor in medicine, not diet, not smoking, not exercise, not stress, not genetics, not drugs, not surgery that has a greater impact on our quality of life, incidence of illness and premature death from all causes."

– Dean Ornish, M.D. (1998) in *Love and Survival*

The Healing Power of Love

Essential Elements Of Love

Love is indeed a many splendored thing! Love is real chicken soup for the well-being of the mind, body and soul. It is valuable for health and yet a free medicine. Love is an almighty power that can cure many maladies. Let us use it for health, happiness, and to achieve longer life (King, 1998). Let us first understand the ten essential elements of love.

1. Understand and know yourself completely and be totally truthful.
2. Be honest and unselfish.
3. Be tender and forgiving, compassionate and sympathetic to others.
4. Accept yourself and love yourself no matter what.
5. Give generously expecting nothing in return.
6. Learn to forgive and forget.

7. Smile and give thanks always.
8. Share everything with everybody, especially with the unwanted, crippled, blind, sick, and dying.
9. Love thy neighbor and other folks.
10. Recognize that the heart and soul have to generate love.

Spousal Love

> *"Love is liking someone better than you like yourself."*
>
> – Frank Tiger

Love should have no boundaries. Love your spouse, children, parents and relatives. Love your neighbors, friends, co-workers, strangers and pets. Remember love develops from emotional togetherness and trust, communication and commitment, friendship and flexibility. Let us look at the act of loving the spouse. The following ten steps should be the elements of total spousal love (Kirshenbaum, 1998):

1. Do all the essential things for your spouse.
2. Keep the promises.
3. Respect your spouse. Avoid belittling words. Treat your spouse as a best friend. Talk freely, openly, fully.
4. Reserve five minutes every day to look continuously at your spouse.
5. Discuss your grievances with your spouse with compassion and sympathy.
6. Solve the problems of the spouse, don't let anyone else be first.
7. Touch, hug, kiss, hold hands, at least once a day. Have good sex. "Love is the poetry of senses." – Honoré de Balzac
8. Always remain together to enjoy the fun activities of life.
9. Support each other, be generous in giving, show you care, be kind.
10. Express your recognition and appreciation for all the good acts of the spouse.

Our prescription: Love everyone, but love your spouse specially.

Love And Longevity

"Love is of all passions the strongest for it attacks simultaneously the head, the heart and the senses."

– Voltaire

Ten facts to prove that love enhances longevity:

1. Love is an important nutrient of the immune system (Bock and Sabin, 1997).
2. Married persons live longer, healthier.
3. Love and intimacy have great powers of healing (Ornish, 1998).
4. Married persons are less prone to injury and disability.
5. Married persons are less likely to have chronic illnesses.
6. Deep emotional relationship reduces incidence of coronary artery disease.
7. Love is an important factor in reducing risk of angina.
8. Love is a great stress buster.
9. Love creates peace and emotional stability.
10. Love promotes sleep.

Our final words: Love must not diminish with age, for love protects you from aging.

References

Bock, K. and Sabin, N. (1997). *The Road to Immunity. How to Survive and Thrive in a Toxic World.* New York, NY : Simon and Schuster, Inc.

Kingma, D.R. (1998). *The Future of Love, The Power of the Soul in Intimate Relationships.* New York, NY: Doubleday.

Ornish, D. (1998). *Love and Survival.* New York, NY; Harper Collins Publishers.

Section VI.

Caring for Your Body: A Systemic Approach to Longevity

Chapter 22

⊰≫ ⊰≫

Caring for Your Body

Your Body Parts and How They Work

In order to protect the whole body one must take steps to care for each individual system. The human body functions maximally if each system performs optimally. Therefore, it is as important to keep all systems healthy as it is to treat a diseased system. Often the health of one system is dependent on the health of others. For instance, if you have a heart attack or stroke, the functions of several other systems will be affected. Maintenance of good health of the whole body is the ultimate key to longevity.

In this chapter, ten systems comprising almost the entire human body are defined as to their components and functions. Ten of the most common diseases in the world affecting each system are mentioned in Table 22.1. Table 22.2 indicates the percentage of elderly afflicted with chronic conditions. This is followed by a list of ten measures to protect each system. The steps are simple. The use of a lot of common sense is involved. You will find this is a simple, sensible, safe and effective way to earn many extra years. The steps are presented to simply make you aware of what needs to be done and what you can do to be healthy and live longer.

The Nervous System: Protect it and Use it

The nervous system anatomically consists of the brain, hindbrain, pons, medulla, spinal cord and cranial and peripheral nerves. The other component of the central nervous system is the "mind." The brain is

TABLE 22.1

Ten Most Common Causes of Death Globally

Cause of Death	Deaths/ Year
Infectious parasite diseases	10,726,000
Diseases of circulatory system	9,676,000
Unknown causes	8,124,000
Cancers	6,013,000
Acute lower respiratory infections	4,110,000
External causes (injuries, etc.)	3,996,000
Perinatal and Neonatal causes	3,180,000
Diarrhea and dysentery	3,010,000
Chronic lower respiratory diseases	2,888,000
Tuberculosis	2,709,000

the boss of the body. It sends messages and directs all the organs in the body. In other words, it orchestrates the functions of every component of the human body. It is the captain of the team that calls all plays. It makes you see, hear, smell, speak, laugh, cry, love, hate, move and feel pain, touch and it regulates temperature. The "mind" as a co-captain deals with the psychological aspects of human behavior. The following are ten common central nervous system problems:

1. Stroke: also called a cerebrovascular accident, is caused by a blockage of the artery supplying blood to the brain or by a bleed (hemorrhage) within the brain. The consequences of a stroke vary. A massive stroke could cause coma and death. Damage to one side of the brain would cause paralysis of the arm and leg

TABLE 22.2
Percentage of People > 65 with Common Chronic Conditions

Chronic Condition	Men	Women
Arthritis	36 %	55 %
Hearing impairment	36 %	25 %
Hypertension	35 %	46 %
Heart disease	33 %	29 %
Limb deformity	14 %	19 %
Cataracts	10 %	21 %
Visual impairment	10 %	9 %
Emphysema	8 %	2 %
Cerebrovascular disease	8 %	5 %
Ulcers	4 %	3 %

on the opposite side. A very minor stroke, which leaves no permanent damage to the brain, is called TIA (transient ischemic attack). This frequently causes some degree of temporary dizziness and imbalance. Arteriosclerosis and hypertension cause these strokes.
2. Alzheimer's disease. This is the disease named after Alois Alexander who described the changes in the brain such as atrophy of the brain, reduced numbers of neurons in the cortex and neurofibrillary tangles in the surviving neurons. Approximately 7-8% of persons over the age of 65 have Alzheimer's disease. No test is available to make a definite diagnosis. Treatment is largely supportive.

3. Depression is an illness that causes suppression of mood, interference with normal functioning and a distinctive change in thinking. It results in low self-esteem, feelings of worthlessness, inadequacy, and uselessness; anorexia, weight loss, sexual dysfunction, constipation, and agitation.
4. Parkinson's disease was first described by James Parkinson in 1817. Tremors are its most common symptom. Its cause is not known. Symptoms appear when about 85% of the substantia nigra is degenerated. Several drugs are being used and more and more are coming on the market.
5. Epilepsy. Epileptic attacks, fits, seizures and convulsions mean the same. Epilepsy may be caused by changes in the brain but sometimes no definite changes are detected. Current methods of treatment effectively control seizures.
6. Dizziness is an important system that may be caused by many different conditions. It may signify critical problems in the brain such as TIA.
7. Injuries to the central nervous system can cause a variety of symptoms including coma.
8. Meningitis. The three bacteria most commonly causing meningitis are Neisseria Meningitis, Hemophilus Influenza, and Streptococcus Pneumoniae. Treatment with antibiotics should be started immediately. If meningitis is caused by Neisseria meningitis, treatment of contacts is recommended.
9. Migraine headaches affect 5–10% of the population. There is no cure for migraine but the headaches responds well to several medications.
10. Insomnia.

Ten ways to protect your central nervous system

1. Keep your mind active. An active mind keeps other systems functioning better and longer. Loss of memory begins at age 30. Keeping the mind active can slow this loss. The active mind of Bertrand Russell allowed him to write the famous *Human Society in Ethics and Politics*, at the age of 82, and Frank Lloyd Wright drew architectural plans of the Guggenheim Museum at the age of 88.

Caring for Your Body

2. Sleep enough. Proper amount of sleep keeps the brain and all other systems functioning better.
3. Avoid nervous system toxins. Chronic, excessive use of alcohol, tranquilizers, marijuana, sedatives and hypnotics will adversely affect brain functions.
4. Control your diabetes. Glucose is an important brain nutrient and appropriate levels will prevent loss of brain cells.
5. Breathe clean air. Brain functioning depends on oxygen. Too much carbon monoxide, nitrous oxide or other toxic gases can damage the brain.
6. Exercise regularly. This will improve the oxygen supply to the brain and invigorate the whole body.
7. Stop the clogging of brain arteries with proper diet.
8. Stop smoking.
9. Build psychological strength. Be positive. Be optimistic. Beat stress.
10. Stimulate your mind. Read, write, play games that are thought provoking.

The Hematologic System: The Juice of Life, Protect It

Hematology is the branch of medicine that deals with diseases of the blood and different factors involved in the formation of blood and clotting factors. The hematologic system consists of blood, bone marrow and lymphoid tissue. Blood is composed of red blood cells, white blood cells and platelets. The red blood cells provide the life line, oxygen, to every part of the body. This oxygen is carried by hemoglobin, which is part of the red blood cell. There are about 280 million molecules of hemoglobin in each red blood cell. The white blood cells are the defenders of the body. These are neutrophils and mononuclear phagocytes made in the bone marrow. Mononuclear phagocytes are versatile in destroying invading enemies, eliminating debris and remodeling normal tissue. Neutrophils simply destroy enemies. The platelets regulate the clotting mechanics of blood.

The most common disorders of the red blood cell system are anemias. Abnormalities of white blood cells cause leukemia. Deficiency

TABLE 22.3

Ten Best Sources of Iron

Daily Requirement:	For Men: 10 mg RE For Women: 15 mg RE
Item	Serving
Beef Liver	3 oz
Clams	3-4 oz
Oysters	1-2 oz
Bagel, Bran Muffin	2
Oatmeal, instant	2/3 cup
Cereal	1 oz
Apricots	1 cup
Peas, Lentils	1 cup
Soy Beans	1/2 cup
Beans	1 cup

of platelets causes problems such as bleeding under the skin. The following are ten hematologic diseases:

1. Iron deficiency anemia.
2. Pernicious anemia (vitamin B12 deficiency).
3. Megaloblastic anemia (folic acid deficiency).
4. Sickle cell anemia.
5. Acute leukemia.
6. Chronic leukemia.
7. Thrombocytopenic purpura.
8. Thrombophlebitis (clots in veins).
9. Hemophilia.
10. Thalassemia.

How can you protect your hematologic system? What precautions should you take? What should you look for? Here are ten prescriptions:

1. Eat a diet with sufficient amounts of iron to prevent anemia (see Table 22.3). If indicated, take iron supplements.
2. Look for foods that are good sources of vitamin B12 to prevent anemia. Vegetables are great.
3. Sickle cell anemia is a genetic condition most commonly seen in African Americans. This segment of the population should get a Sickle Cell screen, a simple blood test. Individuals with the condition will need treatment for anemia and sickle cell crises.
4. Protect your immune system. Treat infections as soon as possible.
5. Don't be fooled by vague symptoms like fatigue, weakness and dizziness. You may think these are caused by the flu but in fact, you may have a hematologic problem. Get checked.
6. If you are diagnosed with hemophilia, take extreme care to prevent injuries. Bleeding could be a serious consequence.
7. Fever and chills after a blood transfusion can be from mismatch of transfused blood. Alert the doctor or nurse.
8. Many medications cause blood disorders. Educate yourself about the medicines you take.
9. If you have a problem with phlebitis (inflammation of the veins) avoid prolonged periods of sitting or lying down. Walk around every so often to prevent formation of clots in the veins. Dislodgment of these clots and their journey into the lungs can be serious.
10. If you have a hematologic condition get regular check ups and blood tests as indicated by your physician.

The Endocrine System: Your Glands, Guard Them

The word "endocrine" refers to the production of biologically active substances in the body. The endocrine glands release these substances, the hormones, into the systemic circulation. The endocrine system consists of several glands that secrete and supply different hormones for a variety of functions. These glands include the anterior pituitary, posterior pituitary, pineal gland, thyroid gland, parathyroid glands, adrenal glands, pancreas, testes, ovaries, prostate gland and breasts. The disturbances in the functions of these glands produce a variety of conditions. Here is a list of ten diseases of the endocrine system:

1. Diabetes mellitus.
2. Hypoglycemia.
3. Hypothyroidism, hyperthyroidism.
4. Addison's disease—deficiency of andrenocortical hormones.
5. Hypertension.
6. Alteration of growth.
7. Sexual dysfunction, infertility.
8. Hirsutism
9. Gynecomastia.
10. Tumors of glands.

As a patient, you can play a part in the diagnosis and treatment of some of the conditions. Think of diabetes if you have a family history of diabetes and have symptoms such as excessive thirst, excessive appetite, tiredness and increased frequency of urination. If you have symptoms of dizziness, tremors and sweating, consider hypoglycemia. Hypothyroidism, an underactive thyroid, is a common condition and may be associated with tiredness, depression, dry skin and hair, puffy face, slow heart beat, cold intolerance, weight gain, constipation and brittle nails. Excessive growth of hair, enlargement of breasts in males and development of any unusual signs or symptoms should alert you to see your doctor. Take the following ten simple steps to come out ahead:

1. Get regular medical check-ups.
2. If you are a diabetic, monitor your blood sugar, get foot care three or four times a year, monitor your blood pressure and get counseling on your diet. At least once a year have an eye examination, cholesterol test, kidney function tests, and get a flu shot.
3. Watch out for rapid weight gain or weight loss. This could be from a thyroid problem.

4. Get menstrual irregularities evaluated. Get a Pap smear once a year.
5. Check your pulse rate and blood pressure periodically. If the pulse rate is slow or fast (normal is 70-80 beats per minute) or the blood pressure is high (over 140 systolic and 90 diastolic) inform your doctor. These changes may be due to thyroid or adrenal gland problems.
6. Do self-examination of breasts once a month to check for lumps.
7. If you have hypoglycemia make sure to stick to high protein, low carbohydrate hypoglycemic diet.
8. Do not abuse drugs, especially cortisones.
9. Reduce stress. This means less adrenaline and consequently a good heart rate, normal blood pressure and a strong immune system.
10. Prevent premature aging of the endocrine system by eliminating obesity.

The Dermatologic System: The Mink Coat

The skin, the biological clothing that we are born with, is one of the body's most important organs. It is a simple organ, consisting of two layers, the outer epidermis and the inner dermis. Within the skin are the sweat and sebaceous glands, as well as blood vessels, nerves and hair.

The skin performs several important functions. The most important and the least talked about function is the physical protection it provides. Imagine the vulnerability of the entire body without this protection! The fitting of this God-given garment holds everything together. Besides these two important functions, the skin protects us against the loss of essential fluids from the body and the entry of microorganisms and toxic agents. It also protects us against extreme environmental temperatures and ultraviolet radiation. The function of the skin is indeed crucial to our survival.

Every system in the body is affected by aging. The skin is no exception. Sun exposure over the lifetime accelerates the aging of skin.

This is reflected in the form of thin, wrinkled skin. The major changes are laxity, wrinkling, uneven pigmentation, infections, and a variety of cancerous and non-cancerous conditions. Here is a list of ten common conditions:

1. Cancers of skin—melanomas and squamous and basal cell carcinomas.
2. Fungal infections.
3. Acne.
4. Contact dermatitis.
5. Drug reactions.
6. Infections—boils, chicken pox, scabies.
7. Eczema and urticaria.
8. Herpes simplex and herpes zoster (shingles).
9. Psoriasis.
10. Keratoses, corns, calluses.

What can you do to best preserve your protective robe? Here are ten tips:

1. Limit your sun worshipping, especially if you are fair-skinned. Use sunscreen preparations. Sun is a major factor in the development of melanoma. About 35,000 melanomas are diagnosed each year in the U.S. About 700,000 cases of non-melanoma cancer a year in the U.S. are sun-related.
2. Eating right can prevent many cancers of the skin.
3. Limit the calories from fat to about 20% of total caloric intake.
4. Consume five servings of fruits and vegetables every day.
5. Eat foods high in Beta-carotene.
6. Get adequate supplies of Vitamin E. It helps to prevent skin cancers.
7. Pay special attention to skin hygiene.
8. Avoid excessive use of tanning parlors.
9. Consult your physician if you see a black lesion developing. This may be a melanoma.
10. Get a periodic skin survey by a dermatologist or your personal doctor.

The Respiratory System: The Breathing Apparatus, Keep it Clean

Oxygen is an absolutely essential commodity without which life cannot be sustained. Your respiratory system is the supplier of this nutrient. This system consists of your mouth and nose, the larynx, trachea, bronchi and your lungs. The lungs are composed of billions of air sacs called alveoli. Here in these sacs is where the inhaled air with oxygen is transferred into the pulmonary capillaries and then into the blood circulation for eventual transport to every part of the body. We cannot allow the ultimate lifeline, the pulmonary system, to malfunction. Don't forget lung disease is the number three killer in America. One or more of the diseases affecting this system will create symptoms such as cough, excess mucus, blood in sputum, shortness of breath, wheezing, chest pain, blue nails and swelling of legs or other parts. Here are ten common conditions:

1. Cancer of the lungs.
2. Bronchitis.
3. Pneumonia, infection of lungs by bacteria, viruses and fungi; influenza.
4. Asthma.
5. Allergic rhinitis (hay fever).
6. Emphysema (chronic obstructive pulmonary disease—COPD).
7. Bronchiectasis, infection and distension of alveoli.
8. Tuberculosis.
9. Sleep apnea.
10. Respiratory failure.

This is what you can do to protect your respiratory system and reduce risk of illness. It is important to emphasize that any malfunction of the respiratory system will adversely affect many other systems in the body.

1. Do not smoke. One in five deaths in the U.S. is smoking-related. The CDC (1997) advises that "quitting smoking has major and immediate health benefits for smokers of all ages. After 10 years off cigarettes, the risk of lung cancer in former smokers drops to less than one-half of that of a continuing smoker."

2. Avoid passive smoking. Second hand smoke causes about 3,000 deaths each year from lung cancer in people who don't smoke.
3. Exposure to asbestos particles and to minerals like silicon, beryllium, and chemicals such as uranium, arsenic, vinyl chloride, nickel chromate, coal products and mustard gas can cause lung cancer. Select jobs where there is no risk of exposure to these substances.
4. Get vaccinated against influenza and pneumonia.
5. Get PPD or Tine test to check for tuberculosis. This is a curable disease.
6. Regular check-ups and chest x-rays are important. Comply with your doctor's orders.
7. If you are coughing up blood see your doctor as soon as possible.
8. If you suffer from asthma, learn to treat acute symptoms and care for chronic asthma (Polk, 1997). Be educated about the use of inhalers and bronchiodilators. For emergency use carry them with you.
9. If you are oxygen-dependent, be fully knowledgeable about the equipment and its use.
10. Keep allergy medicines handy.

The Cardiovascular System: The Ticker System

The heart is a simple pump made of muscle. It is at the center of the cardiovascular system. Unoxygenated or impure blood is brought to the lungs by veins from different parts of the body. The lungs oxygenate this blood and return it to the heart. The heart, in turn, pumps the oxygenated or pure blood out into the aorta, the largest artery of the body. The inflow and outflow of blood is controlled by four valves of the heart. The entire body is supplied oxygenated blood by the branches of the aorta. The first branches of the aorta are the coronary arteries, which supply blood to the heart itself. Thus, the cardiovascular system is similar to a plumbing system with a simple mechanical function of pumping and distributing blood. In a plumbing system the failure of the pump or blockage of one pipe may disrupt the whole system. In the human body the malfunction of the heart or blockage of one of the

Caring for Your Body

arteries, such as a coronary artery may disrupt the functions of all systems. When the cardiovascular system is affected, one may experience one or more of the symptoms like chest pain, palpitations, dizziness, fatigue, shortness of breath and edema. Ten common diseases affecting the cardiovascular system are:

1. Hardening (Atherosclerosis) of the aorta, coronary arteries and peripheral arteries that results in narrowing of the passages.
2. Heart attack (coronary thrombosis with damage to the heart muscle).
3. Hypertension.
4. Enlarged heart (cardiomyopathy).
5. Diseases of the valves (valvular heart disease).
6. Rheumatic fever with valvular heart disease.
7. Irregular heart beats (arrhythmias).
8. Congenital heart disease.
9. Infection of the heart (myocarditis).
10. Congestive heart failure.

The diseases of the heart can affect other organs and the diseases of other organs can affect the function of the heart. In other chapters several aspects of protecting the cardiovascular system are detailed. A list of ten protective steps:

1. Get children checked to rule out any congenital heart defects.
2. Control blood pressure.
3. Exercise regularly.
4. Maintain ideal body weight.
5. Stop smoking.
6. Eat diets with low fat and low saturated fats.
7. Limit total cholesterol intake to less than 300 mg per day.
8. Maintain with exercise, diet and medications blood cholesterol level below 200, triglycerides below 200, HDL cholesterol between 35 and 65, and LDL cholesterol below 130.
9. Treat diabetes.
10. Get regular check-ups.

The Gastrointestinal System: The Food Pipe

"A good set of bowels is worth more to a man than any quantity of brains."

– Henry Wheeler Shaw

This system is just a simple pipeline. It consists of the mouth where food is chewed, the esophagus that carries it to the stomach. Digestion starts there and continues in the duodenum. The small intestine propels forward what is received from the stomach, separating the good stuff that is absorbed in the blood stream, and the bad stuff (fecal matter) that is emptied into the large intestine for final elimination through the rectum.

As you put the food in your mouth, the digestive juices start to work on it. The salivary glands secrete serous ptyalin that initiates the digestive process. The stomach secretes pepsinogen, gastric lipase and amylase to continue digestion which is further helped by the enzymes produced by the pancreas. The intestines, the rhythm house of the body, complete the job of giving the body what is good for it and getting rid of what is not. The rhythm goes on day and night. The faithful work even when we sleep.

One would think that such a simple system should function effortlessly. Not so. We create turbulence and malfunction by what we do—eat the wrong things, ingest undesirable substances and live sedentary lives. We forget that "the fastest path to wellness is through the stomach" (Rosenthal, 1998). We pay the price and end up developing the following ten conditions:

1. Indigestion.
2. Gastroesophageal reflux disease (GERD), acid peptic disease.
3. Gastritis (inflammation of the mucus lining of the stomach).
4. Constipation.
5. Diverticulosis.
6. Hemorrhoids.
7. Carcinoma of the colon.
8. Pancreatitis.
9. Irritable bowel syndrome (spastic colon).
10. Peptic ulcer.

As we get older the gastrointestinal system gets weaker and slower. The glands produce less digestive enzymes, stomach muscle gets sluggish and the intestinal peristalsis slows. Several of the above conditions result from these aging processes. There is a lot you can do to protect your digestive system and minimize the problems. Here are ten tips:

1. Stop indigestion. This can be effectively done by chewing the food well, not eating large meals, eating low fat meals, drinking plenty of water, eating at regular hours and exercising. In short, eat well, live well and feel well. These steps will also stop premature aging of the gastrointestinal system and prolong life.
2. Eliminate reflux. Are you suffering from symptoms of regurgitation, gaseousness, chest pain, heart burn and belching, aggravated by bending or lying down? If you are, chances are you have a gastroesophageal reflux problem. Just remember obesity, smoking, eating fatty foods, caffeine, large meals, alcohol and drugs are the factors predisposing to reflux. Knowing this you know what to do.
3. Extinguish fire in your stomach: Alcohol, aspirin, anti-inflammatory medications, iron, and spicy foods can irritate your stomach lining, increase acid production and inflame the mucosa. This is gastritis. Remove the cause and take antacids for symptom relief.
4. Prevent constipation: common-sense measures are described in Chapter 25.
5. Prevent weakness in the wall of the large intestine. The weakness results in the formation of little blisters in the wall. These blisters are called diverticuli. The wall gets weaker as we age and 50 % of people over the age of 70 have these. Minimize the risk of getting these by eating high roughage food and preventing constipation.
6. Do you want to reduce the misery caused by hemorrhoids? First, prevent them by increasing intake of dietary fiber, forcing a habit of regular bowel movements and preventing constipation. If you have hemorrhoids, use sitz baths and cortisone suppositories.

7. The American Cancer Society has done a lot in the fight against cancer of the colon. For early detection follow their protocol. A great number of cancers of the colon can be prevented with a low fat, high fiber diet. Stick to it, it is good for your heart too.
8. There are several causes of pancreatitis but the one that commonly causes pancreatitis is alcoholism. Eliminate binge drinking.
9. What can you do if you have a peptic ulcer? See your doctor and he will treat the common cause of the ulcer, infection by Helicobacter Pylori. As a patient you can address other causal factors—avoid cortisones, anti-inflammatory drugs, stop smoking and reduce stress.
10. How should you deal with a spastic colon? Understand that it is a mind-body situation; your brain controls the gut. Emotions and stress play a big part. Counseling is the most effective tool in the management of irritable bowel syndrome: "The spirit of dialogue provides opportunities for healing." –Stan Saterem, M.D. You can do a lot for yourself. Don't let spastic colon control you. Pray, meditate, exercise, sleep well and avoid alcohol, tobacco and narcotics. You will soon find out that you have the power to heal yourself.

The Urinary System: The Clearing House

The urinary system consists of the kidneys, ureters, bladder, prostate and urethra. The kidneys are composed of filtering units called nephrons. There are about a million of those in each kidney. As we get older these nephrons gradually get destroyed. It is estimated that by the age of 70 we lose about half of the nephrons. However, this does not endanger life because it is possible to live a perfectly normal life even with one-third of functioning nephrons. All the unwanted filtered waste is transported to the bladder by the ureters. They are removed via the urethra as urine.

The kidneys are "public servants" of the body picking up and hauling away garbage and dirty water. If the kidneys do not function properly the body will become a sewer with unwanted, poisonous water.

This back-up, in turn, will seriously affect other systems. Let us first enlist ten of the most common conditions affecting the urinary system:

1. Arterionephrosclerosis—thickening of the arteries within the kidneys caused by hypertension, diabetes.
2. Pyelonephritis—infection of the kidneys.
3. Renal calculi (kidney stones).
4. Cystitis (infection of the bladder).
5. Prostatitis (infection of the prostate).
6. Carcinoma of the prostate.
7. Carcinoma of the bladder.
8. Carcinoma of the kidney.
9. Acute kidney failure.
10. Chronic kidney failure.

These are several measures one can take to protect the urinary system, prevent some diseases and extend your life span. Here are ten:

1. Drink at least eight glasses of water daily to maintain the filtering function of the kidneys adequately.
2. Diabetes seriously affects the arteries and the glomeruli in the kidneys. Keep blood sugar under control.
3. Hypertension causes thickening of the arteries and can lead to kidney failure. Be compliant with the management of high blood pressure including administration of medications and sodium restriction.
4. Many risk factors for heart disease are also risk factors for kidneys. Prevent atherosclerosis with diet and lifestyle changes.
5. Watch your calcium intake to reduce the risk of kidney stones.
6. Practice safe sex to reduce the risk of infections of the urethra, bladder, prostate and kidneys.
7. Avoid the ingestion of harmful chemicals, including excessive amounts of alcohol.
8. To reduce the risks of prostate cancer, eat a low fat, high-fiber diet with five servings a day of fruits and vegetables and exercise regularly.

9. Take steps for early detection of prostate cancer. Get regular rectal examinations and the blood test for prostate cancer. Fifty-eight percent of all prostate cancers are discovered while still localized and the five-year survival rate for men with localized prostate cancer is 100%. This makes a compelling case for early detection with regular rectal examination and PSA tests.
10. If you notice blood in your urine, contact your physician as soon as possible.

The Musculoskeletal System: The Mobility Machine

The system that gives you the most aches and pains in your body is this system, composed of the muscles and bones. The muscles and bones in the body work whenever we move. With so many spare parts and so many activities it is no wonder that some things go out of gear now and then and we end up with a problem. As we get older, the muscles get more and more tired and the joints show the signs of wear and tear. Consequently, age brings more aches and pains. We all get headaches. And, who does not get a backache? Most of the common symptom-creating conditions in the musculoskeletal system are generally disabling versus fatal. However, disability becomes a significant condition, especially in later life. The disabilities affect the person's lifestyle, family relations, employability and self-image.

These may not kill you but they would cause nagging disability. Here are ten such conditions that commonly affect persons of all ages:

1. Muscle spasms and strains.
2. Backache.
3. Sciatica (inflammation of sciatic nerve).
4. Osteoarthritis and osteoporosis.
5. Rheumatoid arthritis.
6. Bursitis (inflammation of bursa).
7. Tendonitis (inflammation of tendon).
8. Carpal tunnel syndrome.
9. Myalgias (muscle pains).
10. Diseases of spine (e.g. slipped disc, cervical radiculopathy).

The protection of the musculoskeletal system requires two principal considerations: prevention of injury and prevention of disease. Here are prescriptions to safeguard this system:

1. Maintain good posture. This will reduce muscle fatigue and prevent disfiguring and disabling curvature of the spine.
2. Prevent injuries by doing physical activity within the range of power of the muscles and motion of the joints. Go slowly and gradually.
3. Avoid awkward and excessive movements.
4. Avoid chronic trauma. Adopt safe exercises, especially in the older age.
5. Prevent slips and falls. Fractures such as a hip fracture can lead to fatal complications.
6. Choose proper exercises. Weight bearing exercises reduce the risk of osteoporosis.
7. Prevent osteoporosis (bone loss) with hormone therapy. Bone loss begins at about age 40 and accelerates after that. The rate of loss in women is twice that compared to men. Men lose 3% of skeletal weight per decade and women 8%. A bone density study helps estimate the degree of bone loss. Postmenopausal women should consult their physicians to evaluate the need for estrogen (premarin) to slow or prevent osteoporosis.
8. Get enough calcium. Calcium is gradually lost from the bones and the bones become more brittle and more likely to fracture. Everyone, young or old, needs enough calcium. Men and women ages 35–50 need 1,000 mg of calcium per day. After menopause a women needs 1,000 mg of calcium if she is taking estrogen but 1,500 mg if she is not. Get calcium, preferably from dietary sources. Drink a glass of skim milk daily.
9. Get enough vitamin D from diet and sunlight. Older adults who do not get enough vitamin D from diet or sun may need supplemental vitamin D. To assess your needs consult your physician.
10. Sleep on a comfortable, semi-firm mattress to allow your body the best rest at night and the most ideal resting spot to rejuvenate for the next day.

Immune System: The Department of Defense

This is an important system. It consists of lymphocytes and monocytes (white blood cells) circulating in our blood and bone marrow and collected in lymphoid tissue (lymph nodes, spleen, peyer's patches, lymphoid patches in intestines, thymus, tonsils and appendix). What makes these organs part of an army of defenders are the principal cells in B and T lymphocytes and cells of the monocyte-macrophage lineage. These cells and their products, antibodies and lymphokines, provide protective immunity. This immunity is critical for survival of humans in the world of bacteria and viruses. If the system becomes dysfunctional or fails to respond, microorganisms win and disease results. AIDS is a classic example of such a failure.

In a healthy person the basic elements of the immune system work together in a regulated manner and provide rapid, specific and highly protective defenses against foreign invaders. On the other hand a weak immune system can expose us to devastating illnesses. This is why maintenance of a powerful immune system is a passport to good health and longevity.

Just look at the list of the following ten common conditions to appreciate why we need to keep our immune system fit to fight these diseases:

1. Acquired Immune Deficiency Syndrome (AIDS).
2. Anaphylaxis (hypersensitivity reaction).
3. Infectious diseases (caused by bacteria, viruses, and parasites).
4. Asthma.
5. Allergic rhinitis.
6. Insect sting allergy.
7. Drug and food reaction.
8. Contact dermatitis.
9. Rheumatoid Arthritis.
10. Lupus erythematosis.

There is a wealth of information on the immune system and how to boost it. Some of the information is based on sound medical principles and some is conjectural. Let us make it simple. Anything

Caring for Your Body

that is going to keep the human body mentally and physically strong is going to contribute to strengthening the immune system. As we get older we become less active and abuse our body by not eating right. The immune system consequently gets weaker and our defenses falter. To live longer it is vital to keep our "Department of Defense" in good order. The following are ten simple prescriptions to achieve that:

1. Use mind-body power. The endorphins produced by different cells in the body work with the immune system to reduce pain and suffering and improve mood. How do you raise the level of endorphins? It is simple. Laugh, love, forgive, seek self-respect, and happiness.
2. Use the antioxidant armamentarium wisely. You can get just about all the vitamins you need if you choose your foods wisely. Use supplements when indicated.
3. Use the right diet to strengthen your immune system. Carbohydrates are good immune system builders.
4. Use a low fat diet. Fox and Fox (1997) recommend a diet with 20% fat, 10% protein, and 70% carbohydrates.
5. Reduce stress. All the steps to reduce stress and to cope with acute and chronic stress are discussed in Chapter 20.
6. Exercise regularly. Exercises improve your mental and physical health. They help you maintain weight, strengthen your heart, tone your muscles, lower the blood pressure, increase the level of your good cholesterol and overall make you feel better and live longer. See Chapters twelve through seventeen. A study of 17,000 Harvard graduates concluded that the students who burned 2,000 calories per week with exercises lived longer than those who exercised less or not at all (Fox and Fox, 1997).
7. Use your brainpower. The brain can weaken the immune system by leading you into depression, unhappiness, anxiety, irritability and mood swings.
8. Use your spiritual and emotional powers. Develop intimate relationships and a positive attitude. Pray and meditate. Learn to cope.

9. Stay out of harm's way. Refer to the book by Levy and Monte (1997), for good advice on tools to boost your immune system.
10. Be moderate. Avoid excesses. Live a balanced life within yourself and within the world around you.

References

American Cancer Society. (1997). Cancer. Website: http://www.cancer.org.

Braunwald, Isselbacher, Wilson, et al, Eds. (1994). *Harrison's Principles of Internal Medicine,* (13th edition). New York, NY: McGraw Hill, Inc.

Centers for Disease Control. (1997). Smoking. Website: http://www.cdc.gov.

Fox, A. and Fox, B. (1997). *Boost Your Immune System Now.* Rocklin, CA: Prima Publishing.

Levy, E. and Monte, T. (1997). *The 10 Best Tools to Boost Your Immune System.* Boston, MA: Houston Mifflin Company.

Polk, I.J. (1997). *All About Asthma. Stop Suffering and Start Living.* New York, NY: Insight Books, Plenum Press.

Rosenthal, S. (1998). *The Gastrointestinal Sourcebook.* Los Angeles, CA: Lowell House.

Salt, W. B. (1997). *Irritable Bowel Syndrome.* Columbus, OH: Parkview Publishing.

Chapter 23

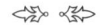

⥽ ⥼

Action Plans for Each of the Ten Decades

We want to increase longevity. We know that if we eliminate major causes of death, we can substantially increase longevity. To do that first we need to know what the common causes of death are. Then we can identify the measures we can take to prevent such deaths in each decade. The approach is simple. Leading causes of death are listed first, followed by recommended interventions to prevent deaths in each decade.

First Decade of Life

The ten leading causes of death:

1. Accidents and adverse effects, including motor vehicle accidents and other accidental adverse effects
2. Congenital anomaly
3. Malignant neoplasms, including lymphatic, hematopoietic tissues
4. Homicide and legal intervention
5. Diseases of heart
6. HIV infection
7. Pneumonia and influenza
8. Perinatal conditions
9. Septicemia
10. Cerebrovascular disease

If these are the leading causes of death, what should you do?

1. Accidents being the most common cause of death in the first decade of life, take the preventive actions.
2. Obtain proper prenatal, perinatal and postnatal care to protect the newborn.
3. Get the child periodically checked by a doctor to evaluate for any congenital abnormalities, signs of infections, malignancies, etc.
4. Immunize the children fully and on time.
5. If the mother is HIV infected, seek medical advice from a specialist.
6. Be informed about Sudden Infant Death Syndrome or crib death to be able to take preventive steps.
7. Limit your children's television watching to a minimum; allow only educational programs, cartoons and sports; control viewing to avoid violent shows.
8. Help children develop healthy eating habits with nutritional foods. Restrict junk foods and soft drinks. Encourage natural juices and water.
9. Do not expose children to passive smoke.
10. Maintain open communication with children and provide emotional support to prevent depression; encourage social involvement with other children and adults.

Second Decade of Life

The leading causes of death for this decade are:

1. Accidents including motor vehicle accidents, and their complications.
2. Malignant neoplasms including lymphopoietic and hematopoietic.
3. Homicide and legal intervention.
4. Congenital anomalies.
5. Suicide.
6. Diseases of heart.
7. HIV infection.

8. Chronic obstructive pulmonary disease and allied conditions.
9. Pneumonia and influenza.
10. Cerebrovascular diseases and benign neoplasms.

The recommended interventions for this decade pertain mainly to children and adolescents. They are:

1. Encourage safe driving by teenagers; demand seat belt use.
2. Teach healthy eating habits and maintain ideal weight.
3. Maintain regular medical checkups; get specialist care for those with HIV infection, congenital anomaly or chronic illness; get pneumococcal and influenza vaccination for high risk individuals.
4. Maintain an open dialogue; discuss relevant issues such as teen violence, sex education, drug abuse; answer questions; watch closely for any signs of depression, change in behavior, change in eating habits.
5. Do not allow children to smoke or subject them to passive smoke (teach them the dangers of smoking).
6. Keep guns out of the house or safely locked up.
7. Do not expose the children to your harmful habits of adults—alcohol and drug abuse, smoking.
8. Discourage excessive television viewing.
9. Encourage physical activities, team sports.
10. Encourage participation in school activities, hobbies; help to develop a positive attitude and self esteem.

Third Decade of Life

The leading causes of death for this decade are:

1. Accidents including motor vehicle accidents, and their complications.
2. HIV infection.
3. Homicide.
4. Suicide.
5. Malignant neoplasms.
6. Diseases of heart.

7. Congenital anomalies.
8. Chronic obstructive pulmonary diseases and allied conditions.
9. Pneumonia and influenza.
10. Cerebrovascular diseases.

The recommended actions and interventions are:

1. Drive defensively; wear seat belts and follow speed limits.
2. Be informed about AIDS and other sexually transmitted diseases.
3. Keep guns out of the house or safely locked up.
4. Maintain regular medical checkups; self breast exam, pelvic examination and pap smear; skin exam every three years; get specialist care if you have HIV infection.
5. Maintain open dialogue with parent or elder peer to discuss issues of violence, sex education, depression, eating disorders.
6. Keep healthy eating habits; avoid alcohol, drugs.
7. Do not smoke or be subjected to prolonged passive smoke.
8. Exercise regularly and maintain ideal weight.
9. Get pneumococcal and influenza vaccine if you are at high risk.
10. Continue participation in group activities, sports to develop positive attitude and self esteem.

Fourth Decade of Life

The leading causes of death for this decade are:

1. HIV infection.
2. Accidents and adverse effects including motor vehicle accidents and other accidents, adverse effects.
3. Malignant neoplasms.
4. Diseases of heart.
5. Suicide.
6. Homicide and legal intervention.
7. Chronic liver disease and cirrhosis.
8. Cerebrovascular disease.
9. Diabetes Mellitus.
10. Pneumonia and influenza.

For this decade you should do the following:

1. AIDS and other sexually transmitted diseases awareness; methods of transmission and prevention; specialist care for those with HIV infection, chronic illness.
2. Drive safely; wear seat belts and follow speed limits. Do not drink and drive.
3. Maintain regular medical checkups as in the previous decade. Maintain strict compliance with all prescribed medications. Do not smoke or be subjected to prolonged passive smoke.
4. Maintain a healthy diet and ideal weight; exercise regularly.
5. Seek treatment for depression.
6. Keep guns out of the house or safely locked up.
7. Avoid alcohol abuse or seek treatment for alcohol or drug abuse.
8. Exercise regularly.
9. Awareness of preventive measures and treatment that can be taken with regard to medical illness with strong family correlation, e.g. hypertension, high cholesterol, diabetes.
10. Pneumococcal and influenza vaccination for high risk individuals.

Fifth Decade of Life

The following are the leading causes of death for this decade:

1. Malignant neoplasms including lymphatic and hematopoietic.
2. Diseases of heart.
3. Accidents and adverse effects including motor vehicle accidents and other accidents.
4. Cerebrovascular disease.
5. Chronic obstructive pulmonary disease and allied conditions.
6. Diabetes Mellitus.
7. Chronic liver disease and cirrhosis.
8. HIV infection.
9. Suicide.
10. Pneumonia and influenza.

Then what should you do for this decade? Here is simple advice:

1. Maintain regular medical checkups; obtain screening mammograms every year, self breast exam (women) every month, get a screening pelvic exam and pap smear every year: may be less if three consecutive negative examinations, wear sunscreen, get skin examination every three years.
2. Maintain a healthy diet and ideal weight. Exercise regularly. Check cholesterol, fasting blood sugar yearly. Be knowledgeable about family history.
3. Drive safely; wear seat belts and follow speed limits. Do not drink and drive.
4. Maintain strict compliance with all prescribed medications. Get checked if you have headaches, dizziness, unsteadiness.
5. Do not smoke or be subjected to prolonged passive smoke.
6. Be informed about diabetes, get regular check ups, blood sugar checks, eyes and feet examinations.
7. Avoid alcohol and drugs and/or seek treatment for drug or alcohol abuse. Get treatment for depression.
8. AIDS and other sexually transmitted diseases awareness; methods of transmission and prevention; specialist care for those with HIV infection, chronic illness.
9. Keep guns out of the house or safely locked up.
10. Pneumococcal and influenza vaccine for high risk individuals. Ophthalmologic examinations to assess need for glasses.

Sixth Decade of Life

The leading causes of death for this decade are as follows:

1. Malignant neoplasms, including lymphatic, hematopoietic.
2. Diseases of heart.
3. Accidents and adverse effects, including motor vehicle accidents and other accidents.
4. Cerebrovascular disease.
5. Chronic obstructive pulmonary disease and allied conditions.

Ten Action Plans For Each Of The Ten Decades

6. Diabetes Mellitus.
7. Chronic liver disease and cirrhosis.
8. HIV infection.
9. Suicide.
10. Pneumonia and influenza.

If these are the leading causes of death, this is what you should do:

1. Maintain regular medical checkups and get tests as above plus yearly fecal occult blood test and a digital rectal examination and prostate specific antigen test for males and flexible sigmoidoscopy every three to five years.
2. Follow a heart-healthy diet and maintain ideal weight. Exercise regularly. Check cholesterol, fasting blood sugar yearly. Be knowledgeable about family history.
3. Drive safely and defensively; wear seat belts and follow speed limits. Do not drink and drive.
4. Maintain strict compliance with all prescribed medications. Get checked if you have headaches, dizziness, unsteadiness.
5. Do not smoke or be subjected to prolonged passive smoke.
6. Be informed about diabetes, get regular check ups, blood sugar checks, eyes and feet examinations.
7. Avoid alcohol or drug abuse and/or seek treatment.
8. AIDS and other sexually transmitted diseases awareness; methods of transmission and prevention; specialist care for those with HIV infection, chronic illness.
9. Keep guns out of the house or safely locked up.
10. Follow all of the above steps.

Seventh to Tenth Decades of Life

The leading causes of death in these decades are:

1. Diseases of heart.
2. Malignant neoplasms, including lymphatic and hematopoietic.
3. Cerebrovascular diseases.
4. Chronic obstructive pulmonary disease and allied conditions.

5. Pneumonia and influenza.
6. Diabetes Mellitus.
7. Accidents and adverse effects, including motor vehicle accidents and other accidents.
8. Alzheimer's disease.
9. Nephritis, nephrotic syndrome and nephrosis.
10. Septicemia.

So what are the things you should do? Here is a short summary:

1. Maintain a healthy diet and ideal weight. Exercise regularly. Check cholesterol, fasting blood sugar yearly. Be knowledgeable about family history.
2. Maintain regular medical checkups; self breast exam, pelvic examination and pap smear; skin exam every three years; get specialist care if you have HIV infection.
3. Maintain strict compliance with all prescribed medications. Get checked if you have headaches, dizziness, unsteadiness.
4. Do not smoke or be subjected to prolonged passive smoke.
5. Pneumococcal and influenza vaccine for high risk individuals. Ophthalmologic examinations to assess need for glasses.
6. Be informed about diabetes, get regular check ups, blood sugar checks, eyes and feet examinations.
7. Drive safely; wear seat belts and follow speed limits. Do not drink and drive.
8. Do everything to prevent falls, burns, etc.
9. Get evaluated and treated for fevers, chills, swelling of legs, shortness of breath, chest pains, dizziness and weakness.
10. Follow all of the above steps.

Chapter 24

Beating the Major Killers

Our action plans have identified the leading causes of death for each decade and clarified many of the things you can do in each decade to increase longevity. But, what are the most major concerns and what can you do? Here is a short list of tips to help you combat the most common major killers.

i. Heart Disease: The Common Killer, Prevent It

This is how you do it:

1. Be informed about heart disease.
2. Be aware of family history.
3. Get regular check-ups including checks for cholesterol, HDL, LDL, triglycerides and glucose.
4. Do not smoke.
5. Treat high blood pressure and diabetes.
6. Eat heart-healthy.
7. Exercise regularly.
8. Prevent obesity.
9. If you have signs or symptoms such as chest pain, shortness of breath, irregular pulse, palpitations, leg swelling; consult a physician.
10. Discuss chest x-ray, EKG, echocardiogram, stress test and angiogram with your physician. Refer to chapters on diet, exercise, smoking and obesity for more information.

ii. Conquer the AIDS Virus

Here are ten ways to do it:

1. Understand the cause, methods of transmission and means of preventing this infection. HIV is spread by sexual transmission and contact with infected blood. By practicing "safe sex" with use of barrier precautions, not breast feeding if infected and avoiding shared needle use with intravenous drug abusers, there is decreased likelihood of contracting infection.
2. Recognize the gravity of the problem. 42.3 million people have been infected with HIV since the start of the epidemic. More than 12 million people have died as a result. In the United States, HIV infection/AIDS is the second leading cause of death among adults ages 25-44 (CDC, 1997).
3. To stay healthy longer, heed the following recommendations if you are infected with HIV:

    - Go to a physician who is aware of the latest in HIV/AIDS treatment and follow his/her instructions, keep appointments, take medications.
    - Get immunized to prevent common infections like pneumonia and the flu.
    - Don't smoke or use drugs, eat healthy foods, exercise regularly.
    - Get enough sleep and rest, take time to relax, ease stress.

4. Take antiretrovirals. By taking these medications, those with HIV can slow their progression to AIDS and death (CDC, 1997).
5. For early diagnosis of HIV infection, obtain counseling if:

    - You consider yourself at risk for infection.
    - You are of childbearing age as infection can be spread to the infant.
    - You are attending sexually transmitted diseases and drug abuse clinics.
    - You are seeking family planning services.

- You are the sexual or needle-sharing partner of an injecting drug user.
- You have tuberculosis.
- You received blood transfusions or blood component transfusions between early 1978 and 1985.
- You are an immigrant entering the U.S.

6. Be involved with research to find a cure. Contribute financially. Participate in studies if you are infected.
7. If you are pregnant and HIV positive, remember mother to child transmission can be greatly reduced by taking antiretroviral medication throughout the pregnancy and by giving it to the infant for several weeks after birth.
8. Get tested. There are numerous anonymous testing sites, home tests are available and physicians are capable of referring for testing. From the time of possible exposure, there can be a delay of three and rarely even six months before a positive test. It is advised to have repeat testing at three and six months after a possible exposure.
9. Take advantage of educational programs.
10. Be aware, AIDS can be conquered. Prevent new infections.

iii. Accidents Kill, Stop Them

These are the ways to save lives:

1. Drive defensively—wear seat belts, do not drive if you drink alcohol, follow speed limits.
2. Ensure proper safety measures to prevent falls.
3. Install pool and lake fences to prevent drowning.
4. Keep guns out of the house or safely locked up.
5. Keep medications, detergents and poisonous chemicals out of reach of children.
6. Enforce use of safety gear such as helmets, pads for children riding bikes and skating.

7. Install safety measures at the workplace.
8. Buy safe, age-appropriate toys for children to prevent choking, falls, suffocation and burning.
9. Take steps to prevent fires.
10. Keep electrical system well maintained and cooking gas containers properly secured.

iv. Improve the Odds Against Cancer

The national medical organizations have developed a consensus on how to prevent cancer. You will be taking the very best steps if you follow the counsel in the following short summary which is based on the works of these organizations. Recognize the cancer toll. Cancers cause hundreds of thousands of deaths and reduce overall longevity.

1. Lung cancer: Do not forget, one death out of every five in the U.S. is smoking related; the CDC (May 23, 1997) indicated that every year smoking kills more than 278,000 men and 152,000 women. When you smoke, everyone around you smokes. Passive smoking kills about 3,000 people in the U.S. yearly. Therefore, do not smoke. If you are a smoker go for regular check ups, chest x-rays and try every method to quit.
2. Breast Cancer: Take the following steps to prevent breast cancer or to detect it early:

    - Monthly self breast examinations after age 20.
    - Breast examination by your physician, age 20-40, every three years and over 40 every year.
    - Mammograms for women age 40 and over, every year.
    - Breast ultrasound as recommended by your physician. Sometimes the lumps seen in the mammogram are not well defined. To separate a cyst from the tumor, breast ultrasound becomes necessary.
    - Biopsy of the lump if recommended by your physicians.

3. Get rectal examinations and PSA test for early detection of prostate cancer as follows: Digital rectal examination and PSA annually beginning at age 50. For men in high risk groups (family history) digital rectal examination and PSA beginning at age 45. Undertake a prostate ultrasound and/or biopsy as recommended by your physician.
4. Colon and rectum cancer: For early detection the following protocol is recommended for men and women over 50:

    - Fecal occult blood tests every year and a flexible sigmoidoscopy every five years or colonoscopy every ten years, or double contrast barium enema every five to ten years. All these procedures should be accompanied by a digital rectal examination. Consult your physician if you are a high risk patient with a family history of colon and rectum cancer.
    - Sigmoidoscopy and digital rectal exam every five years.
    - Or colonoscopy and digital rectal exam every ten years,
    - Or double contrast barium enema every five to ten years, plus digital rectal examination

5. Cancers of the cervix, uterus and vagina: To prevent these, women should follow the prescribed schedule of examinations and pap smears as follows:

    - Pap test and pelvic examination for sexually active women over age 18 every year. If three consecutive normal results, may do less frequently.
    - Women at high risk should have endometrial tissue biopsy when menopause begins.

6. Skin cancers: Skin cancers are extremely common . Over one million cases of skin cancer are diagnosed each year in the United States are considered related to exposure to the sun. Protect yourself with sunscreens, umbrellas and shelters. Other cancers with direct environmental factors: Overuse of alcohol can increase the risk of cancers of the mouth, larynx, throat, esophagus,

breast, liver; smokeless tobacco (chewing tobacco or snuff) can increase the risk of cancers of the mouth, larynx, throat and esophagus; estrogens used for menopause may increase the risk of endometrial carcinoma; and radiation and exposure to chemicals like benzene, asbestos, vinyl chloride and arsenic can increase the risk of cancer. Take proper steps to reduce these risks.
7. Cancer and your food: The right foods can reduce the risk of developing cancer. To beat the odds of cancer the American Dietetic Association (1998) recommends the following dietary formula:

- Low fat, high grain products with vegetables and fruits.
- 6–11 servings of bread, cereal, rice and pasta.
- 2–4 servings of fruit or fruit juice.
- 3–5 servings of vegetables.
- 2–3 servings of low-fat or nonfat milk, yogurt; and
- 2–3 servings of lean meat, skinless poultry, fish, eggs, dry beans, or nuts.

The vitamins C, E and beta carotene are also important in reducing the risk of cancer. Get generous supplies of vitamin C from oranges, grapefruit and citrus juices and vitamin E and beta carotene from whole grain breads and cereals, green leafy vegetables and fruits.

8. Final prescription to reduce the risk of cancers: stop smoking, eat the right foods and follow medical protocols. By following this simple advice, millions of deaths will be prevented and millions will live longer.

v. Obesity is a Disease, Trim It

1. Prevent obesity.
2. Determine appropriate calorie needs and eat within the limit of calories needed.

3. Limit total calories from fat to less than 30 percent.
4. Snack sensibly.
5. Avoid all-you-can-eat places.
6. Exercise to lose weight.
7. Pay special attention to a sedentary lifestyle—move, move, move. Don't be a couch potato.
8. Trim teenage obesity by cutting television watching (JAMA, 1998).
9. Keep fruits and water in the refrigerator instead of chips and soft drinks.
10. Follow the five steps to success for losing weight. For more details refer to Chapter 19.

vi. Hypertension: The Silent Killer, Control It

1. Be aware of family history of hypertension.
2. Get regular check-ups.
3. Be compliant with medications prescribed.
4. Get urine examination and kidney function tests—BUN and creatinine.
5. Get chest x-ray to check for possible enlargement of heart caused by hypertension.
6. Salt (sodium) plays a part in your blood pressure problem, take in what is recommended, avoid excesses.
7. Relaxation techniques, stress control, exercise are important factors in blood pressure control. Review the chapters on exercise and stress reduction.
8. If you have uncontrolled high blood pressure, seek the opinion of a nephrologist.
9. The higher the weight, the higher the blood pressure. Control weight to control blood pressure.
10. Watch out for the symptoms and signs of hypertension, such as shortness of breath, dizziness, headache, and swelling of legs. Go get checked by your doctor.

vii. Do Yourself and Others a Favor: Don't Light Up

Smoking cigarettes leads to nicotine addiction. This addiction leads to effects spanning all decades. Lung cancer, heart disease and emphysema are all effects of smoking. The effects of secondhand smoke are evident in causing illnesses even among those who do not smoke themselves, such as children living in a house with smokers.

Cigarette smoking is the main cause of preventable lung cancer (Harrison, 1994). It increases risk of coronary artery disease, stroke, pneumonia, bronchitis and emphysema and smoking during pregnancy decreases oxygen supply to the fetus, increasing risk of spontaneous abortion and fetal death. Stopping smoking provides benefits regardless of how long you have been smoking. Help yourself and others by not smoking. For details see Chapter 18.

viii. Suicides: Prevent Them

As you can see from the causes of deaths in different decades, suicide ranks among the top ten in every decade. The Institute of Mental Health (1996) reports that in all age groups, there are 10.8 suicides per 100,000 persons and in the age groups of 15–24 there are 12 suicides per 100,000 deaths. The CDC reports that 25,000-30,000 deaths per year are suicides (CDC Website, 1994). There are 100 to 120 suicide attempts for every one suicide death. This equals 1.3% of all deaths. An alarming fact is 50% of all suicides are committed with firearms. Some suicides are committed by drugs, drowning and a combination of alcohol and drugs.

Many of the suicides are preventable. If the psychological and psychiatric problems of the adolescents and young adults are recognized early and proper intervention is provided, deaths of many young people can be prevented. The society should wake up to the problem of the troubled ones. Besides providing psychological help, the means to commit suicides should be addressed. Easy access to guns, alcohol and drugs should be eliminated. With serious efforts, there will be fewer suicides causing a significant impact on longevity.

ix. Murder Mania: Cure It

In 1994 there were 23,730 murders, according to the CDC. In the age group of 14–17 years, 7.3 deaths among 100,000 persons were from murders. This number rises to 19.2 deaths out of 100,000 persons in the age group of 18–24 years. After the age of 25, the number of homicidal deaths drops to 6.4 per 100,000 persons (Bureau of Justice, 1997). The gun, again, is responsible for the majority of murders. Domestic arguments with or without the use of alcohol and drugs is also a significant factor. Are we a sick society? In the U.S., murder ranks number four in the first decade of life, number three in the second and third decades, and number six in the fourth decade. It is obvious from these data that we lose a large number of our young people through criminal killing. Nowhere in the world are the numbers so high.

The murder mania has a lot to do with the easy availability of guns but also the psychological frame of our society. Education on violence prevention, treatment of the psychologically disturbed and strict gun laws would make a significant difference. None of us should just stand by and do nothing.

x. Influenza and Pneumonia: Don't Wait, Vaccinate

1. Pneumonia is one of the leading causes of death, and in many instances, especially in the elderly population, it is preventable by vaccinating against specific viruses and bacteria. Influenza and streptococcus pneumonia are two such infections.
2. Influenza virus causes the flu which accounts for numerous visits to emergency rooms and doctors' offices. Oftentimes hospital-

ization is required for complications of this viral illness. The number of hospitalizations per year is approximately 130,000 to 170,000. The aim of influenza vaccination must be to prevent complications especially in those people that are considered high risk.
3. Target groups for influenza vaccination:

- Persons older than 65,
- Residents of nursing homes or chronic care facilities,
- Adults and children with chronic lung or heart disease,
- Adults or children with illnesses such as diabetes mellitus, kidney problems and blood disorders,
- Women who will be in their second or third trimester of pregnancy during the influenza season,
- Children 6 months to 18 years of age who require long-term aspirin therapy,
- Health care professionals caring for high-risk patients,
- Household contacts of high-risk patients.

The time for vaccination is mid-October to November to prevent illness during flu season, which is from December to March (CDC, 1997).
4. Streptococcus causes ear infections, pneumonia and meningitis. It is responsible for approximately 40,000 deaths annually. This accounts for more vaccine-preventable deaths than any other bacterial infection. Despite appropriate antibiotic therapy once a blood infection is diagnosed, the death rate of this illness is 15-20 percent among high risk adults. Thus, the importance of vaccination in disease prevention is paramount.
5. Remember pneumonia vaccination is recommended for:

- Persons older than 65
- Persons with chronic heart or lung diseases or diabetes,
- Persons with no spleen, or spleen dysfunction,
- Immunocompromised people with HIV or cancers,

- Persons with alcoholism, chronic liver disease or sickle cell disease,
- Persons with renal failure, nephrotic syndrome Hodgkin's disease, myeloma.

6. The safety of vaccinations has been well established. However, there have been reported side effects. These include soreness at injection site, fever and sometimes mild symptoms resembling viral influenza. Physicians giving you the vaccination will review any possible side effects with you.
7. Sometimes re-vaccination may be required. Consult your physician to find out when and why you need re-vaccination.
8. Immunization recommendations can change.
9. Current recommendations are included in Table 3 in the appendix.
10. For the latest information, contact your doctor or the local health department, because the recommendations may be changed with the changing onslaught of the diseases.

Our final word: Vaccinate. In less than one minute, you buy long-term protection from a disease that can kill you.

References

American Cancer Society. (1997). Prevention and detection guidelines. Website: http://www.cancer.org/guide.

American Dietetic Association. (1998). Website: http://www.eatright.org.

Braunwald, Isselbacher, Wilson, et al, Eds. (1994). *Harrison's Principles of Internal Medicine,* (13th edition). New York, NY: McGraw Hill, Inc.

Centers for Disease Control. (1997, May 23). Website: http://www.cdc.gov.

Centers for Disease Control. (1994). Website: http://www.cdc.gov.

Centers for Disease Control Division of HIV/AIDS Prevention. (1997). Website: http://www.cdc.gov.

Cowley, C. (1998, November 30). Cancer and diet. *Newsweek*, 60-66.

Institute of Mental Health. (1996). Website: http://www.nimh.nih.gov.

Relationship of physical activity and television watching with body weight and level of fatness among children. (1998). *Journal of the American Medical Association, 279*, 938-42.

United States Department of Justice. (1997). Website: http://www.ojp.usdoj.gov.

PART II

Prescriptions for Longevity: The Best Practices

Chapter 25

❖ ❖

100 Prescriptions to Live to Be 100

I. Caring for Your Body

i. Be Educated About Your Brain And Body

Your brain and body are your most valuable assets. Your sense of well-being stems from their proper care and maintenance. Only when you understand what your body and brain are and how they function, can you learn how to care for yourself. Chapter 22 has prepared you to take steps towards achieving better physical and mental health and a longer life.

ii. The Brain: Use It Or Lose It

The human brain contains over 100 billion nerve cells and billions of other types of cells. It is estimated that we lose about 100,000 brain cells every day and by the age of 50 about two billion cells die. Once the brain cells are dead they are lost forever; they do not regenerate.

The brain is exceptionally vulnerable to insults as a result of hardening of the arteries, strokes, diabetes, immune diseases, infections, respiratory insufficiency, abuse of alcohol and drugs. Good nutrition, exercise and pursuit of peace through prayers, meditation, biofeedback and love maximize the brain function. Prevent diseases of all other body organs to protect the brain. The general cannot survive without protection from the army.

Anything you don't use rusts or degenerates. The brain is no exception. Samuel Johnson said: "It's a man's own fault, it is from want of use if his mind grows torpid in old age."

Involve yourself in brain stimulating activities. Read books, newspapers, magazines, write, debate, play chess or cards; do crossword puzzles; play stocks; learn a new word every day. Think about the people who have done it.

iii. Avoid Brain – Body Poisons

A majority of Americans indulge in excesses. The teenagers and younger adults abuse marijuana, amphetamines, cocaine, heroin, LSD and many other mind-altering drugs. The abuse of alcohol by teenagers and adults is rampant. People overuse even prescription drugs such as sleeping pills, psychotherapeutic agents as well as hundreds of over-the-counter medications. Over the counter drugs and prescribed medications kill more than 100,000 Americans and seriously injure an additional 2.1 million every year (Lazarou, et al, 1998). It has been pointed out in Chapter 9 that vitamin supplements are often used unnecessarily. Excessive indulgence in the use of many of the dietary items including sodium, fats, proteins and carbohydrates is extremely common. The soft drinks are no exceptions. All these excesses affect the brain and many systems of the body in different ways. Be prudent. Be wary of untested products.

iv. Beware of Quacks, Ads and Fads

Quackery is defined as promotion of false or unproven health claims for profits and quacks are the people who sell unproven medications. Don't be brainwashed by them. They may promise a quick fix or a cure for cancer. They may provide simple conclusions from complex studies or derive conclusions based on a single study.

The dangers of quackery are harmful effects from items sold, and delay in getting legitimate treatments. Longevity buffs get fooled by quacks with powers of advertising, promises of quick, easy, safe, effective treatment, and baseless guarantees.

What is advertised as "natural" or "safe" is not necessarily good for your health. Rely on scientific facts and not on the advertised claims. Don't be a victim of misleading ads, fads and claims.

v. Beat Depression

The following are common symptoms of depression:

- Lack of energy and motivation and impaired concentration.
- Feelings of being sad, low, blue and down in the dumps and being agitated and irritable.
- Despair with feelings of hopelessness, worthlessness and guilt.
- Poor appetite, loss or gain of weight and constipation.
- Lack of interest in daily activities and lack of interest in sex.
- Crying spells and suicidal ideation.
- Impaired concentration, slow thinking and forgetfulness.
- Indecisiveness and ineffectiveness.
- Mood swings, listlessness and fatigue.
- Sleeping problems.

If your problem is a minor one, you can help yourself by taking the following ten steps:

1. Engage yourself in mind-occupying activities: read, write, play with the computer.
2. Socialize—visit your friends, co-workers, relatives, and neighbors.
3. Express your feelings to whomever you think is your well wisher and do not hesitate to ask for help.
4. Exercise—play sports, go for walks, swim. Do things with others.
5. Watch comedy shows on television and avoid sad stories.
6. Do not seek solace in alcohol or drugs as these may increase your depression.
7. Involve yourself in prayers with people. Go to church, synagogue and pray and talk to people.

8. Develop new hobbies, do volunteer work, occupy yourself, and stay busy.
9. Get good sleep.
10. If those measures fail, do not hesitate to seek the services of your physician or a psychotherapy professional.

Our prescription: If your problem is a serious one, seek professional help.

vi. Prevent Constipation

If the frequency of your bowel movements is fewer than two per week, by definition, you are constipated. Constipation creates a very nagging feeling: the mind feels uneasy, the body feels out of gear. The result is a very uncomfortable state of existence with gas and bloating. Constipation is a nasty disease.

Perhaps the most important cause of constipation is poor evacuatory habits. In a rush to get to work in the morning many people neglect to attend to nature's call. When this becomes a recurrent ritual, constipation becomes a costly complication.

Another significant factor is the lack of physical activity, which causes slowing of intestinal mobility. Depression, anxiety and stress contribute to constipation. In our pill-popping era, many of us use and abuse pain killers, antacids and psychotherapeutic drugs. These contribute to the creation of chronic constipation. Laxatives are over-used. Frequent use of laxatives leads to abandonment of prudent preventive measures.

A common outcome of constipation is hemorrhoids. The condition called diverticulosis (formation of pouches in the wall of the intestine) is often associated with constipation. The risk of cancer of the colon is also increased with the occurrence of chronic constipation.

When constipation is a reality, the simplest medical measures are the use of high fiber diet, the use of a stool softener such as Colace or about two teaspoons of Metamucil with fruit juice. Soften the stools to prevent constipation with at least eight glasses of water every day. Chew food well before swallowing to improve digestion as well as render the stools soft. Regular walking reduces the incidence of constipation by promoting peristalsis and improving advancement of intestinal contents.

Our prescription: Heed nature's call and invest the necessary amount of time on the commode.

vii. Prepare for the Sunset Years

Your body needs greater care and attention as you get older. Your loved ones may not be around. You may suffer from disabilities. Your finances may fall short of your needs. You may end up at the mercy of government plans that may not be responsive or satisfactory. In short, you may lose the independence to take care of yourself as you wish. This is the reason why you must take steps continuously over decades to prepare yourself to take care of your body in your sunset years. Here are some ways to do it.

1. Avoid money blues. Develop financial independence with financial planning and savings. Save steadily: collect enough to meet your needs.
2. Work as long as possible. Don't let inactivity age you.
3. Prepare for and adapt to life's transitions.
4. Use all the information in this book—stay fit.
5. Maintain physical, spiritual and mental youth. Refuse to get old.

viii. Change Careers, But Don't Ever Retire

A lot is written about retiring (Smith and Smith, 1999). We want to write about not retiring. The idea of retiring, specifically, retiring at age 65, was born in 1935. In that year, the Social Security Act established the retirement age of 65. George Burns once said, "Retirement at sixty-five is ridiculous. When I was sixty-five I still had pimples." He also asked, "How can you live to be 100 if you stop living at 65?" Retirement, indeed, takes a lot out of life:

1. Retirement is not helpful for longevity; it accelerates aging.
2. It has been proven that right after retirement there is a higher degree of stress and a higher death rate. It is like being fired from a job.
3. One of the greatest tragedies of retirement is the waste of talent and productivity it creates.

4. Retirement promotes physical inactivity and overeating. Both are major factors in reducing longevity.
5. Retirement creates mental sluggishness; it takes away a lot of thinking power.
6. Many people lapse into depression after retirement.
7. Retirement creates worry; if you don't work you will have eight more hours to worry about.
8. Retirement robs you of economic power and turns you into an economic liability.
9. Retirement cuts you off of social interaction with co-workers and creates loneliness.
10. Retirement brings boredom.

Think that 65 is just a number with no significance. Think that you can contribute to our society at any age. For yourself, recognize the fact that the right to earn a livelihood does not end at a fixed age. Reassure yourself that you don't get old at 65, you don't lose the capacity to work, you don't lose sexual prowess, you don't get senile or decrepit and you don't lose the ability to think and be productive. If you need a booster, derive inspiration from people who have not retired, aged well and who have continued to be creative, constructive and productive well beyond the age of 65. Think about Grandma Moses who kept painting until her death at 100 and Nobel Peace Prize winner, Mother Teresa who kept working hard helping the poor until she died at age 87. Remember Frank Lloyd Wright kept working as an architect until he died at age 91, George Bernard Shaw kept writing until he died at age 94 and pianist Arthur Rubinstein presented a concert at Carnegie Hall at 89.

Your prescription: Change careers if necessary but don't retire. By not retiring you extend your youth and put the aging process on hold.

ix. Listen to the Health Organizations

The major medical organizations are the true guardians of the human health. They objectively discuss the positives and negatives of the issues and treatments. They develop consensus on all matters that affect your health. Here is a summary of what they do (for more information, all of these organizations can be reached via the Internet):

1. The American Medical Association (AMA): Promotes the art and science of medicine for the betterment of your health.
2. The American Dietetic Association (ADA): Your link to nutrition and health professionals.
3. The American Heart Association (AHA): Helps to ensure the beat goes on…longer.
4. The American Diabetic Association (ADA): The sugar experts.
5. World Health Organization (WHO): Works internationally to help all peoples attain the highest level of health.
6. The American Cancer Society (ACS): Helps us prevent and treat cancers.
7. The American Lung Association (ALA): We breathe better with their help.
8. The United States Department of Health and Human Services: Protects the health of all Americans.
9. The Centers for Disease Control (CDC): Promotes health and quality of life by preventing and controlling disease, injury and disability.
10. The Environmental Protection Agency (EPA): Protects your health by keeping the environment clean and safe.

x. Stop Abusing Your Body

Many diseases are self-inflicted. Various chapters in this book discuss a host of conditions that clearly result from abuse of the body. Overeating causes obesity and several accompanying complications, smoking causes respiratory problems and cancers, stress increases blood pressure, eating the wrong foods results in heart problems, lack of exercise ages you faster, alcoholism leads to liver, heart and stomach problems, and certain supplements result in side effects—just to mention a few of the causes of the difficulties we create for ourselves. Careful consideration and utilization of the following prescriptions and the information in the preceding chapters will help you stop abusing your body.

II. Ten General Medical Prescriptions

i. Get Regular Medical Check-Ups

James Fixx, the author of the best-selling book, *Running*, dropped dead while running at the age of 51. Apparently he had no medical check-up for a long time before he died. Thousands of people die every day, suddenly and unexpectedly. Many have no idea of the extent of their medical problems because of the lack of medical check-ups and millions die prematurely because they fail to have needed check-ups.

There are many medical conditions that are not only detectable but correctable. Without medical check-ups, they could remain undiagnosed and cause unexpected death. Another significant reason for regular medical check-ups is to detect serious conditions that will cause early death if not treated. An apparently healthy person should ideally undergo a routine complete medical check-up every five years up to the age of 30, every three years between the ages of 30 and 49 years, every two years between the ages of 50 and 60 and every year after the age of 60. The purposes of check-ups are to (a) diagnose a medical problem, (b) treat a medical condition, and (c) discuss preventive measures.

Our prescription: Prevent or delay death with medical check-ups.

ii. Comply With Medical Advice

Total compliance with medical advice is important. Non-compliance of the patient is a major problem in medical practice. Often it results in worsening of a medical problem or premature death. Patients show non-compliance in the following ways:

1. Failure to keep appointment.
2. Failure to take prescribed medications.
3. Self-treatment with medications not prescribed by the doctor.
4. Changing dosages without consulting the doctor.
5. Stopping medication without informing the doctor.
6. Not heeding ancillary advice on matters like diet, exercise and smoking.

7. Failure to stick to advice on weight maintenance.
8. Failure to get the recommended special tests such as x-rays and mammograms.
9. Failure to get blood, urine and stool tests, and pap smears.
10. Failure to accept a certain treatment recommendation such as a biopsy or removal of a mass, performance of a procedure or administration of a medication.

Our prescription: The doctor has done his job, now you do yours. Comply with his advice.

iii. Don't Look For Longevity In A Pill Box

Don't pop pills unnecessarily: Think about what is good for you. Millions of prescriptions are written everyday by physicians for their patients. A large number of undesirable situations result in harmful effects from those prescribed drugs. They may be the result of lack of care on the part of the physician, pharmacist or patient. For the ultimate safety of patients, the following ten aspects of drug therapy should be carefully considered by physicians, pharmacists and patients: contraindications, warnings, precautions, adverse reactions, drug interactions, care in prescribing, care in dispensing, overdose, reporting of drug reaction, and immediate treatment to reaction.

Don't pop pills that you really don't need. Take only prescribed medications; take only in doses recommended at times indicated. Report any side effects to your physician as soon as possible.

Every year prescription drugs injure 1.5 million people so severely that they require hospitalization and 100,000 die; making prescription drugs a leading cause of death in the U.S. A study published in *The Journal of the American Medical Association* revealed that, excluding deaths resulting from prescription errors or drug abuse, 106,000 people died from adverse drug reactions in hospitals in 1994 (Lazarou, et al, 1998).

Over–the-Counter Drugs (OTC Drugs): Americans visit their doctors for one-tenth of their health problems. For the rest of the problems they resort to no treatment or self-treatment. Seventy percent of

Americans self-medicate with over-the-counter drugs (see Table 25.1). Americans use more over-the-counter products than people do in other countries.

No drug is completely safe. The over-the-counter drugs are no exceptions. Medical misadventure can result from use of these drugs improperly. Ten causes of such misadventures are as follows (Physician's Desk Reference for Nonprescription Drugs, 1998):

1. An inappropriate medication.
2. An inappropriate dosage.
3. Contraindicated medication.
4. Drug-drug interactions.
5. Side effects.
6. Poor comprehension by user.
7. Vision and hearing impairment.
8. Accessibility to children.
9. Use during pregnancy and nursing.
10. Old age.

Billions of dollars are spent on vitamins, minerals, herbs and "miracle" medicines. Most of them don't improve your health or prolong your life. It has been clearly pointed out that about all of the vitamins and minerals can be obtained from foods. For appropriate indications, refer to the chapter on "Magic Bullets".

iv. Beat The Odds Of Bad Family History

Your grandparents, parents or their siblings may have conditions that can predispose you to medical problems. How do you beat the odds of a bad family history affecting you? Here are ten ways:

1. First be aware of what you have inherited. Know your parents' medical history and history of the siblings of your parents.
2. Certain lifestyle patterns such as alcoholism, violent behavior or smoking may be passed on to you. Prevent or modify these.
3. High cholesterol levels and heart attacks run in families. Get checked at an early age, obtain treatment or change your diet patterns.

TABLE 25.1
Top Ten Complaints of People Using Over-the-Counter Drugs

Complaint	Percentage of People Using an OTC Medication
Headache	76 %
Athlete's foot	69 %
Lip problems	68 %
Common cold	63 %
Dandruff	59 %
Premenstrual	58 %
Menstrual	57 %
Upset stomach	57 %
Painful/dry skin	56%
Sinus problems	54 %

4. Allergies such as rhinitis, eczema, asthma, and dermatitis are present in people who have a family history of these. Prevent symptoms of these by carefully cleaning the house regularly, shampooing the carpet, cleaning drapes, where dust may settle.
5. Rheumatoid arthritis is seen four times as often in people who have a first degree relative who is affected. The benefit of knowing about a family history can lead to early diagnosis and treatment.
6. Lactose intolerance: Prevent the symptoms by using dairy products that are supplemented with the enzyme.

7. Sickle cell disease is a genetic disorder. Genetic counseling among two people who carry this genetic trait is a means of prevention.
8. Certain cancers caused by genes run in families. The risk of breast cancer in a person with a first degree relative (sibling, parent, children) with this cancer is three times the normal risk. Screening mammograms may be advised differently for early diagnosis.
9. As many as 25% of people with colon cancer may have a family history. Earlier age for screening tests such as sigmoidoscopy are recommended in people with this risk factor. Early diagnosis is the best hope for total cure.
10. Diabetes runs in families. Those with a family history may be able to prevent diabetes from occurring by preventing obesity, exercising and following an appropriate diet.

v. Carry Emergency Medicines With You

There are some conditions which require constant attention and timely use of prescribed medicines. The following situations require special treatment.

1. Coronary artery disease with angina: Always carry the nitroglycerin pills with you.
2. Asthma: An asthmatic attack can flare up unexpectedly; carry the inhaler and other medications prescribed by your doctor.
3. Chronic Obstructive Pulmonary Disease (COPD): Many adults with emphysema, lung fibrosis, suffer from shortness of breath. Some are dependent on oxygen. Others manage the problem with bronchodilators. Make sure of your needs and carry bronchodilators, oxygen, etc. with you as prescribed. Many need them every day.
4. Diabetes Mellitus: Patients who are on diabetes pills should carry them along for prescribed use. In addition they should carry candies with them just in case they get an attack of hypoglycemia (low blood sugar). People who are insulin-dependent must, of course, carry insulin with syringes and candies.
5. Blood clotting problems: Some patients who have conditions of clots in the veins, pulmonary embolism (clots in the lungs) or

atrial fibrillation require the use of coumadin. Carry coumadin, an anticoagulant, to prevent formation of clots in the veins, and take it as prescribed.

6. Allergies: Acute allergy symptoms, allergic reactions and acute allergy-induced asthma attacks require immediate treatment. Carry an Epi-pen, which is a syringe with epinephrine that can thwart the attack.
7. Diarrhea: If you are planning to visit foreign countries, it is a good idea to carry Pepto Bismol and a prescription for Cipro 500 mg tablets to be taken as prescribed.
8. Vomiting: A prescription of Compazine from your doctor will help you if you have bouts of vomiting on a trip. If you are planning a boat trip, get a prescription for a patch called TransDerm Scop to prevent sea sickness.
9. For headaches or fever carry aspirin, Ibuprofen or Tylenol.
10. If you are going to be away for more than one day, don't forget to carry all the prescribed medications that you are supposed to take on a daily basis.

vi. Prevent AIDS

There is no cure for HIV/AIDS. Prevention is the only means of staying disease-free. Here are ten ways you can prevent it:

1. Do not have sexual relations with an infected person that would result in contact with semen, vaginal secretions, blood or body fluids.
2. Ask about the sexual history of current and past sex partners.
3. Ask about any history of intravenous drug use.
4. Always use a condom from beginning to end, during any type of sex (vaginal, oral, anal). Use latex condoms rather than natural membrane or lambskin. Latex condoms offer greater protection against sexually transmitted diseases.
5. Do not share needles. Intravenous drug users who share needles may be exposed to HIV as blood may remain on the needle resulting in an exchange.
6. Avoid deep kissing. It may result in abrasions or in people with oral ulcers, there may be possible blood exposure.

7. Avoid sharing toothbrushes or razors, as there may be blood exposure to these items.
8. If you are going to have a tattoo, make sure of the sterility of the items used in the procedure.
9. If you need a blood transfusion, obtain blood from a known family member or friend as opposed to local hospital donations.
10. Be informed; get up-to-date information and answers from the Centers for Disease Control National AIDS Hotline at 1-800-342-2437.

vii. Beat the Five Big C's: Cancer Prevention Protocols

The American Cancer Society (ACS) recommends general cancer-related check-up every three years for people aged 20-40 years and every year for people ages 40 and older. To beat the five big C's note the following guidelines.

Lung Cancer: Get general check-ups as above. Do not smoke cigarettes. Get evaluated if you have complaints of chronic cough, shortness of breath or you are coughing up blood

Breast Cancer: Women age 40 and older should have mammogram, annual clinical breast examination and monthly self breast examination, ages 20-39 should have clinical breast examination every three years and do a monthly self breast examination.

Prostate Cancer: From age 50, get prostate-specific antigen blood test and digital rectal examination.

Colon and Rectum Cancer: Men and women aged 50 or older should follow one of the following: fecal occult blood test and flexible sigmoidoscopy every five years or colonoscopy every ten years or a double-contrast barium enema every five to ten years. All should be accompanied by a digital rectal examination. Higher risk patients should consult their physician about the need for additional testing.

Cervical and Endometrial Cancer: Cervical—all women who are sexually active or who are 18 years or older should have an annual pap smear and pelvic examination. Tests may be done less frequently if three normal consecutive examinations. Endometrial—women at high risk should have an endometrial tissue biopsy when menopause begins.

viii. Breathe Right: Your Lungs are the Lifeline to All of Your Organs

Here are steps you can take to prevent many respiratory problems:

1. Have children vaccinated with H. Influenzae vaccine to reduce infections.
2. Get yearly influenza and periodic pneumococcal vaccines to reduce the bouts of flu and pneumonia, respectively, in later life or earlier depending on your medical condition.
3. Clear the environment of offending allergens to minimize asthma attacks.
4. Stop smoking: 95% of lung cancers are caused by cigarette smoking.
5. Use respiratory protective equipment if you work in places where you are exposed to fumes, asbestos and silica.
6. Join the crusade for environmental protection to reduce the levels of pollution emitted from automobiles or factories.
7. Avoid breathing in secondhand smoke.
8. Get a tuberculosis screening test.
9. Consult a physician as soon as symptoms such as wheezing, shortness of breath, blood in sputum occur, to get the earliest and thus most effective treatment.

The ultimate prescription: Use oxygen, the ultimate lifeline well, by breathing right, for a healthier and longer life

ix. Immunize Children Fully

Childhood immunizations are needed to prevent children from dangerous, possibly life threatening diseases. The diseases that can be prevented by vaccination are:

1. Poliomyelitis that can cause paralysis and even death.
2. Diphtheria that can cause lung infection, heart failure or paralysis.

3. Tetanus that can cause neurological disease.
4. Pertussis which causes whooping cough. It can also cause encephalitis and pneumonia.
5. Measles can cause a contagious rash, lung infection and even fatal encephalitis.
6. Mumps can cause fever, headaches and swelling of cheeks.
7. Rubella (German measles).
8. Hemophilus influenza type B can cause meningitis, pneumonia, blood infection and arthritis.
9. Varicella (chicken pox).
10. Hepatitis B which can cause chronic liver damage.

Immunizations should begin directly after birth and be completed throughout childhood as per recommended schedules. For the current recommended childhood immunization schedules, refer to Appendix A, Table 1.

x. Prevent Falls

About 30% of the elderly fall each year and falls are the sixth leading cause of death in this population. Falls are also the leading cause of nonfatal injuries in older people in the U.S. (Klag, et al, 1999). The elderly and those taking care of them can eliminate many falls. Here are ten tips:

1. Correct the environmental factors. Improve lighting, remove folding and sliding rugs, eliminate slippery areas.
2. Choose even, lighted and safe areas for outdoor walking.
3. Make alterations to ensure the stairs and bathtubs are safe. Choose a one-story residence.
4. Get gait training and improve physical stability.
5. Treat arthritis.
6. Correct vision problems—get proper glasses, treat cataracts.
7. Buy good shoes; use a walking stick if necessary. Walk with a companion.
8. In case of deafness, use a hearing aid.

9. Get treatment for low blood pressure, dizziness, low blood sugar.
10. Eliminate drowsiness caused by use of drugs. Don't risk walking if impaired by drugs or alcohol.

III. Some Diet Prescriptions

i. Learn The Right Ways To Eat: Red Flag Bad Habits

A young man walks into a fast food restaurant and gobbles up a double hamburger, large serving of French fries and a large soft drink in less than ten minutes. The word "fast" is supposed to apply to fast service. It does not mean you have to eat fast. Big bites and quick swallows are common. We have seen in hundreds of autopsy cases totally unchewed chunks of meat and other items in the stomach.

We took a ride in a sight seeing boat, which took us to a spot for a shrimp and ribs dinner. We sat across from a man and his wife; each weighed about 300 pounds. We were simply amazed to see them rushing through dozens of ribs each and mounds of shrimp. It does not take a genius to figure out how they were shortening and destroying their lives. What are the right ways to eat? Here is a list of ten things to do:

1. Eat three meals a day.
2. Avoid non-stop snacking between meals and avoid excessive amounts of soft drinks and desserts. Drink plenty of water.
3. Eat when you are hungry and stop eating when you are full.
4. Eat slowly; allow at least half-an-hour for a meal.
5. Do not eat on the run, while driving or while watching television.
6. Chew the food completely before you swallow.
7. Do not take the next bite before the previous bite is swallowed.
8. Think in advance about your eating strategy if you are attending a dinner party, going on a cruise or visiting a restaurant.
9. Get a dieting companion for better discipline in eating.
10. Make a habit of reminding yourself about the right ways to eat.

Our prescription: Follow the right ways to eat to increase your life expectation. Red flag bad habits.

ii. Eat A Good Breakfast: A Wealth Of Wisdom

Breakfast = A pivotal, life-prolonging meal.

A healthy breakfast—fruits, grains and a glass of milk or orange juice—is important. A good meal first thing helps the body and brain work better throughout the day. Commit yourself to eating a healthy breakfast every day, to help you grow older more gracefully! Here are ten foods you can incorporate into a healthy breakfast, many are things easily found in almost every refrigerator:

1. Fresh fruits, such as apples, peaches or bananas, or citrus fruits such as grapefruits or oranges.
2. A plain bagel, toasted, with low fat cream cheese.
3. Cereal, either cold or hot, with low fat milk.
4. Whole-grain foods, such as bread, bran muffins or rice cakes.
5. Fruit juices, such as grapefruit juice, apple juice or orange juice.
6. Some pastries, such as croissants, but try to avoid sugary foods such as danishes and doughnuts.
7. Scrambled eggs, made from egg whites, mixed with low fat cheddar cheese.
8. Turkey bacon.
9. An English muffin with fruit preservatives (not jelly!).
10. Waffles topped with fruit.

Our prescription: Breakfast. Don't skip it. Get at least 20% of daily calories from this important meal.

iii. Follow The Food Pyramid: Eat For Tomorrow

The Food Pyramid is the best food choices with regard to calories, fat intake, cholesterol, sugar, sodium and alcohol.

1. The Pyramid is an outline of what to eat each day. It calls for eating a variety of foods to get the necessary nutrients and right number of calories. It emphasizes foods from the five major food groups, with the idea that foods in one group cannot replace those in another. This is not a rigid prescription, but a general guideline.

2. The Food Pyramid (see Diagram 1) is made up of the following levels and the number of recommended servings of each (see Chapter 6):
   - fats, oils, sweets (use sparingly)
   - milk, yogurt, cheese and meat, poultry, fish, dry beans, eggs, nuts (2–3 servings of each)
   - vegetables (3–5 servings) and fruits (2–4 servings)
   - breads, cereals, rice, pasta (6–11 servings)

3. The USDA provides the following guidelines for caloric intake requirements:
   - 1,600 calories for sedentary women and older adults
   - 2,200 calories for children, teenage girls, active women and sedentary men
   - 2,800 calories for teenage boys, active men and women

4. Serving regimens:
   - Fats—recommended to limit fat in your diet to 30% of calories with saturated fats to 10% of calories.
   - Cholesterol—Limit the amount of cholesterol intake to average of 300 mg or less per day.
   - Sugars—Limit the amount of added sugar.
   - Salt and sodium—you do not have to give up salt, but limit the amount to no more than 2,400 mg per day. Avoid adding extra amounts.

5. Milk, yogurt and cheese—provide proteins, calcium, vitamins and minerals.
6. Meat, poultry, fish, dry beans, eggs and nuts—supply protein, B vitamins, iron and zinc.
7. Vegetables—provide vitamins A and C, folate and minerals such as iron and magnesium. They are low in fat and also provide fiber.
8. Breads, cereals, rice and pasta (grains) provide complex carbohydrates (starches) which are an important source of energy. They also provide vitamins, minerals and fiber.

9. Alcoholic beverages provide little or no nutrients, but have a lot of calories. See Table 25.2 for the amount of calories in different types of alcohol. Alcohol intake should be in moderation.
10. Take a hike up the Food Pyramid and live longer.

iv. Fight The "Free Radicals" And Win: Eat A Lot Of Vegetables And Fruits

So how can we best safeguard ourselves against the damage that free radical molecules cause? One way of neutralizing free radicals is through antioxidants, which are contained in the vitamins A, C and E and are found in fruits and vegetables. The foods, both fruits and vegetables, that are high in the antioxidant vitamins are: apricots, bananas, oranges, grapefruit, cantaloupe, tomatoes, leafy vegetables, avocado, cauliflower, and carrots.

Our prescription: Eat plenty of fruits and vegetables to fight the "free radical rascals."

v. Follow the Tips About Vitamins and Minerals

Americans spend billions of dollars every year on vitamins and minerals despite the fact that they can get all the vitamins and minerals they need from a wide variety of foods. Nutrient imbalances and toxicities are less likely to occur when nutrients are derived from foods. Most nutrient toxicities occur through supplementation of vitamins and minerals.

Some vitamins and minerals are indicated and medically recommended. Refer to Chapter 9 for details. Here are some important reminders. Fruits, vegetables, grains and beans are excellent sources of vitamins and minerals. The details are in the tables in this book. If you are planning to use vitamins or minerals, consult your physician to determine if you really need them.

vi. Challenge Heart Disease: Eat Heart Healthy

The American Heart Association's principal steps to prevent cardiovascular diseases include smoking cessation, blood pressure control, maintenance of low cholesterol levels, exercise and weight control.

TABLE 25.2
Calories in Alcohol

Alcoholic Beverage	Serving Size	Approx. Calories/Serving
Beer, regular	12 oz	150
Beer, light	12 oz	95
Liquor, 86 proof (gin, rum, vodka, whiskey, scotch)	1.5 oz	90-120
Wine, red	4 oz	85
Wine, white	4 oz	80
Champagne	4 oz	80
Sherry	2 oz	85
Bloody Mary	5 oz	120
Martini	2.25 oz	135
Manhattan	2.25 oz	140
Gin & Tonic	8 oz	180
Screwdriver	8 oz	200

The many aspects of heart disease prevention have been discussed in previous chapters. Here is the summary of those discussions. The dietary and other guidelines for healthy American adults as recommended by the American Heart Association and nine health organizations and government agencies include (AHA, 1997):

1. Nutritionally adequate diet.
2. Loss of excess weight and maintenance of healthy weight.
3. Regular exercises.

4. Diet low in cholesterol, fat, saturated fatty acids. Cholesterol intake less than 300 mg per day.
5. Carbohydrates from fruits, vegetables, whole grains and legumes should provide 55% to 60% of total calories.
6. Smoking cessation.
7. Control of blood pressure.
8. Moderation in use of alcohol.

Dean Ornish pioneered the concept of reversing coronary atherosclerosis. The initial studies indicated that intensive lifestyle changes caused regression of coronary atherosclerosis after one year. He has detailed his studies in his book (Ornish, 1991). More recently he published results of the follow up study (Ornish, 1998). Thirty-five persons were subjected to intensive lifestyle changes (10% fat, whole foods vegetarian diet, aerobic exercise, stress management training, smoking cessation, group psychotherapy support) for five years. The results demonstrated more regression of coronary atherosclerosis after five years than after one year.

vii. Drink Lowfat Milk

Bones need calcium for strength and growth. Only 10% of the nation's elderly persons get the amount of calcium they need and three out of four women do not get enough of it. Lack of calcium can lead to osteoporosis. Vitamin D also aids in the absorption of calcium. Not drinking enough milk can also deprive the body of Vitamin D.

Lowfat and skim milk on the market, plus lowfat yogurt and other products are good sources of calcium and vitamin D. Here are ten suggestions for getting more milk and milk products into your diet to get enough calcium and vitamin D.

1. Drink two glasses of milk a day. That will provide enough calcium to meet the recommended daily amount.
2. Eat a bowl of cereal with skim milk.
3. Eat some lowfat yogurt.
4. Take medications with milk.
5. Mix some lowfat cottage cheese with fruit, and eat it as a snack.

6. Drink a glass of milk with at least one of your daily meals, along with a glass every morning.
7. For a treat, have some lowfat ice cream.
8. For a snack, eat some cheese. There are a variety of lowfat cheeses available at the grocery store.
9. Resist the urge to drink sodas and other drinks without nutritional value, and drink some milk instead.
10. Just like brushing your teeth everyday, make it a habit to drink milk. If all else fails, drink chocolate milk!

Our prescription: It's not hard to keep your bones healthy, milk will do it.

viii. Accept the Bonus From Nature: Gobble Up Fiber

Fiber is good for you. Soluble fiber helps control blood cholesterol levels and insoluble fiber acts as an intestinal cleanser and stool softener. Soluble fibers are pectin and gums. Good sources of soluble fiber are apples, oats and barley. Wheat bran, whole grains and fresh raw vegetables contain insoluble fiber. Other sources of dietary fiber are whole-grain flours, brown rice, fresh fruit, dried prunes, nuts, salads, lentils and peas. Here are ten great ways to get the right amount of fiber:

1. Eat both soluble and insoluble fiber from a variety of different foods.
2. For high fiber, pick popcorn, fresh fruit, fresh raw vegetables and nuts.
3. For breakfast, choose a food with five or more grams of fiber per serving, e.g. bran cereal, oatmeal, whole-wheat muffins or waffles, and fruit.
4. Pick whole-grain products: bread (cornbread, cracked wheat bread, oatmeal bread, whole-wheat bread), cereals, buns, bagels, and pasta. See Table 4.6 for the ten best grain sources.
5. The best fiber source – legumes. Eat two to three times a week.
6. Everyday eat at least five servings of fruits and vegetables.
7. Eat fruits and vegetables with the skin on.
8. Prefer whole fruit to juice.

9. Add high-fiber ingredients (whole-wheat flour, bran) to cooking.
10. Buy items high in fiber—bran, whole-grain and whole-wheat flour. Check labels for fiber content.

Our prescription: "Fiber Up." More fiber means less cholesterol and less constipation.

ix. Drink At Least Eight Glasses Of Water Per Day

In his book, *Your Body's Many Cries for Water*, Fereydoon Batmangelidj (1997) states, "The most important life-giving substance in the body, and the one the body desperately depends on, is water." Although water has no food value, you cannot survive without it. It is an essential nutrient and your health depends on it. It keeps the brain hydrated and regulates the condition of nerve impulses. It is also important for regulation of body temperature, digestion, and elimination of waste from the digestive tract as well as for the maintenance of the immune system (Johns Hopkins Family Health Book, 1999).

Water carries nutrients, hormones and antibodies to and from cells. The body normally loses about two cups of water via breathing, two cups via pores in the skin and about six cups through gastrointestinal and urinary tracts. To replace the loss, the body needs one quart of liquids every day. A loss of one percent or more of total body fluids results in dehydration. Excessive loss of water can occur in hot and humid weather when you perspire a lot, when you have diarrhea or fever and when you exercise. For normal functioning, drink eight glasses of water but drink more if you are losing a lot. It is recommended that you drink more than eight glasses of water if you are suffering from a viral or bacterial infection, constipation or bladder and kidney infections. Do not substitute with tea, coffee, soda or alcohol.

x. For Medical Conditions, Stick to Prescribed Diet Regimens

Diet plays a critical role in our lives. Chapters 4-8 are devoted to various aspects of diet. Inappropriate diets can contribute to the development of new medical conditions or worsen existing ones. On the other hand, proper diets can greatly contribute to improving certain medical problems. Food can be used as medicine. This is clearly outlined in Chapter 8. Ask your physician for advice on diet for your specific problem. This advice is similar to a prescription for a medicine. Stick to the prescribed diet and it could earn you some extra years.

IV. Exercise Prescriptions

i. Eliminate Excuses For Not Exercising

Everyone has excuses for not exercising. Here is a list of ten of the most common excuses and how to deal with them:

1. Too tired: When you work long hours and come home you have a headache, the body feels lethargic and the legs feel rubbery. These symptoms should be the very reason for exercising. Exercise will eliminate these symptoms.
2. Too busy: Nothing should be more important than your health and well being. You can always find time to exercise if you really want to.
3. Too hot outside: Then exercise indoors. This can be done with or without exercise equipment. Swim if you have a pool.
4. Too cold outside: Again, exercise indoors or wear appropriate clothes and get out. Exercise will warm you up and you will find that exercising in cold weather is a lot more fun than watching television, and far healthier.
5. Traveling or on vacation: If you are traveling and staying in a hotel, find the indoor exercise room. Most hotels have facilities for exercises. Most cruise liners have exercise equipment or a swimming pool.
6. Raining or snowing outside: Stay in and exercise. Do spot jogging or use the equipment.
7. Exercise equipment, bicycle broken down: Get it repaired as soon as possible. Until then use the alternatives–walking, jogging, swimming, etc.

8. Street unsafe, park too far, gym too expensive: You can exercise anywhere and everywhere in and around your home. You don't have to spend money on a gym. Most people pay hefty membership fees and don't take full advantage of the facility. Use your own amenities.
9. Exercise buddy away: No problem, do it alone as long as the buddy is away. Adjust to changes in circumstances and circumvent them.
10. Will exercise tomorrow: Don't be a quitter, even for a day.

Our prescription: Don't forget exercise promotes health and longevity.

ii. Exercise Without Exercising

It has been shown that moderate physical activity by sedentary adults for 30 minutes daily yields substantial health benefits (Pratt, 1999). If you have an exercise schedule follow it. Beyond that there are many day-to-day activities that will help you to burn off some of the calories. When you are involved in these activities you don't even know that you are exercising. Here is what you should do:

1. When you go to a store or a mall, park as far away as possible from the shop. If you are in a mall walk around window-shopping.
2. Play with children, grandchildren: Pick them up, walk with them, run with them, play ball games with them, swim with them.
3. Walk your pet: Play frisbee with the dog.
4. Do sit-ups. jumping jacks or use the treadmill while watching television.
5. Attend picnics and use walking trails, and join in sporting activities.
6. Do gardening, mow the grass, and rake the leaves.
7. Clean windows; vacuum carpet; clean garage, driveway and sidewalks; wash the car, clean the pool.

8. Ride a bicycle in the neighborhood; walk for a short distance on errands.
9. Avoid elevator or escalator, instead use stairways.
10. Go dancing.

iii. Choose Safe Exercises

Review Chapters 11–16, which present a broad range of exercises. Whichever activities you choose, keep in mind these ten ways to exercise safely.

1. Check with your doctor before beginning any exercise program, especially if you are over age forty or have risk factors for heart disease.
2. Warm up and cool down. A 5–10 minute warm-up of gentle stretching and light jogging, for example, prevents strains and sprains by increasing muscle elasticity. It also prevents the shock to your system brought on by a rapidly increased heartbeat. A cool down for the same amount of time, meanwhile, prevents the shock of coming to a too-sudden stop.
3. Use safe machines. If you buy a treadmill, be sure it has a low-impact deck to cushion the shock of your activity without jarring your muscles
4. Work out with a buddy especially if you are exercising outdoors or have health problems.
5. If you have arthritis, start exercising at a low level of intensity for short periods of time.
6. If you have asthma, do not work out on those days when your symptoms flare up. Avoid outdoor activity when the air pollution or pollen count is especially bad. If you suffer symptoms during a workout, stop immediately and use your inhaler.
7. If you have diabetes, check your blood sugar level before your workout. If it is under 70 mg/dl, or if you exercise more than one hour after eating, eat something light before beginning your workout.

8. Use appropriate equipment. Buy shoes designed for your sport. And bicyclists, wear a helmet.
9. Drink plenty of water or an electrolyte-replacement drink before, during and after you work out.
10. If you do get hurt, you may ice down the area for 15-20 minutes three times a day for the first one to two days. Use any non-steroidal anti-inflammatory drug. When the pain subsides, take hot showers. After that, try some gentle stretching. Finally get back into exercising slowly. If the injury appears serious or the pain does not ease, make sure to see a doctor.

iv. Choose The Right Place To Exercise

Walking, jogging or bicycling: Most of us can find a place that is relatively free from exhaust fumes, traffic, bad weather and muggers. That perfect location may be a local schoolyard, a shopping mall, an office building (where you have many stairs), or, if necessary your own home. Buy a pedometer and measure how many times around your house you need to walk to make a mile. You will be surprised how easy it is especially with a CD player and an air conditioner!

Turn a room in your house into a permanent or temporary gym with just a few small changes. Purchase an exercise mat for stretches and sit-ups. Buy appropriate exercise equipment. Exercise in an air-conditioned room or at least in one with a fan. And be sure to have ready access to fluids. Finally, if your house is too small or otherwise unfit, arrange to work out at a friend's home gym.

Gyms or health clubs tend to inspire people to work out because they usually require a significant monetary investment. If you go this route, be sure to check out a few before making your selection. Before committing yourself, look for personalized attention and professional expertise. You will also want to be sure that your fitness instructor has proper certification from a nationally recognized certifying organization. Sit or jump in a few classes before you make up your mind. In addition, be sure that you feel at home. Is the club a pick-up spot or a place where muscle-bound men muscle you off the machines? Also, make sure that the equipment is inspected for safety and is of high quality to absorb shock and not to break down in mid-workout.

As you can see, 'no place to work out' is no excuse for not getting exercise.

v. Stretch Here, There and Everywhere

In Chapter 12, we detailed various aspects of stretching. Let us remind ourselves that stretching is just pure fun and good for physical and mental health. Stretching is cost-free, does not require any equipment and it can be done anytime, anywhere. You can begin the day with stretching in bed (see information on stretching exercises in bed in Chapter 12) and stretch all day long at home or at work (refer to information on stretching exercises for the executive). You can stretch from bedroom to bathroom, from living room to family room, from kitchen to patio and anywhere else indoors and everywhere outdoors. No one minds if you stretch in the office, in the malls, on the streets or on the beaches. No one will mind if you stretch in the planes, buses or trains. And, of course, you start with stretching when you get in water (see Chapter 16).

vi. Warm Up, Cool Down

In order to maximize the benefits of exercise, it is vital to prevent injuries and to proceed in a manner that is most natural for the body. Warming up the body prior to intensive exercise and then allowing the body to cool down are, therefore, important. A warm-up is slow, rhythmic exercise of muscle groups done before an activity, to provide the body a period of adjustment time between rest and activity. The American Council of Exercise recommends a warm-up of at least five to ten minutes. This will allow for better overall exercise performance. By slowly involving the muscle groups to be used in exercise, you will help decrease the soreness that may be felt after exercise. Intense work out without any warm-up can lead to early fatigue.

What happens during the warm-up period? There is an increase of blood flow, nutrients and oxygen to the muscles being exercised. This decreases the chance of injury to the muscles and allows joints to work through a maximum range of motion without injury. Warm-up exercises can include walking, slow jogging, knee lifts, arm circles or trunk rotations. These exercises allow low intensity movements of the muscle groups that may be used during more intense exercise.

Cool down involves stretching after exercise to allow muscle relaxation. The muscles need to get back to the normal length. There is also removal of unwanted waste products generated by the body during exercise, such as lactic acid, which leads to the feeling of muscle fatigue. By allowing time to remove these products, the body can then return to its normal state, without the feeling of fatigue. During cool down, your breathing and heart rate should start returning to normal.

Cool down can include stretching leg muscles by side to side lunges, touching toes, arm stretches by reaching behind the back with one arm and holding it with the other. Walking, slow jogging and arm or trunk rotations are also beneficial. Spend about five to ten minutes for the cool down period.

vii. Meet Basic Exercise Requirements

Let us live longer with exercises. Chapters 11–16 have prepared you to exercise. You know what to do. Just start. But before you do, make sure you take all the steps to prepare yourself. Here are the final ten tips.

1. Get evaluated by your doctor to make sure your body is fit and ready for the exercises you want to undertake.
2. Wear appropriate clothes and shoes.
3. Warm up for five to 10 minutes.
4. Select right environment and weather.
5. Do stretching exercises.
6. Exercise within the limits of your body's abilities.
7. Spend five to 10 minutes to cool down.
8. Make safety a must requirement.

9. Be informed about all the benefits of exercises.
10. Exercise discipline and be consistent.

viii. Swim: Water Exercises are Nice and Easy

Do you remember all the benefits of water exercises we presented for you in Chapter 16? What needs to be stressed is that all these benefits come with so much fun. You spend most of the day on ground and so this new medium provides instant excitement of change. When you get in water you automatically move and the movements do not require much effort. The movements involve almost all parts of the body. Your muscles relax and your joints feel good. Your skin cleanses, your heart and lungs get a workout and your mind feels refreshed. You put calories on fire in water. Swim in water if you can. Stretch and workout. Look at all the diagrams in Chapter 16 and you will realize how easy water exercises can be. No sweat, all joy.

ix. Walk, Walk, Walk: Will Be Habit Forming

Walking promotes a long, healthy life. It helps keep joints and muscles in the pink. It helps ensure that your heart is ticking along smoothly. It assists in weight control and overcoming insomnia. It fosters feelings of self-confidence and well-being. And it does much more as you learned from Chapter 13. Then why not rejuvenate the body and mind?

You can walk in the morning, at lunch time afternoon or evening. Walking at any time will render results. Morning walks get your muscles started and your brain going. Those deep breathing exercises between the bursts of walking will oxygenate you for added energy. And the faster ticking of the heart will get this pump in gear for the long haul.

Many of us who go to work experience an afternoon slump. You can bump out this slump by taking a walk at lunch time. Just take a stroll close to work or use a mall.

A brisk walk after work will eliminate your headache, energize your body and put the spring back in your life. Walking gooses your heart, boosts blood flow and delivers oxygen to the cells in the body. The extra heat walking creates in your body will trigger better sleep.

If you walk on a regular basis, you will develop one of the best addictions you can have. If you miss a day, your body and mind will let you know that something is amiss.

x. Don't Slow Down Or Give Up

> *"Is it too late? Ah, nothing is too late till the tired heart shall cease to palpitate."*
>
> -Longfellow

We need to maintain a constant level of exercise to keep our bodies humming smoothly. And the older and busier we get, the harder it is to make exercise a priority.

People who did not work out until their forties, fifties or sixties, can still cut their risk of dying from heart disease and other ailments. Even moderate exercise can make you live longer regardless of your genetic or family history. Try these ten ways to keep the exercise habit:

1. Find a workout buddy. Even if one does not feel up to getting to the gym or track, chances are good that the other one will. And it is harder to let down someone else than yourself.
2. Get a dog. Even if you do not go far, simply taking your pet out for its business twice a day gets you moving.
3. Find an activity that does not feel like work. Choose from dancing, tennis, swimming, walking, aerobics, karate, etc.
4. Choose variety. Switch to another activity; then switch again.
5. Get a good looking outfit and the appropriate shoes, racket or goggles, and you will be more likely to enjoy working out.
6. Spread your exercise days throughout the week
7. Keep a record of your progress. Whether it is a journal of your measurements, repetitions, weight or time, you will find keeping records gives you an added incentive to get out and play.
8. Set personal goals and keep trying to outdo yourself.
9. Promise yourself a treat whenever you reach a goal.
10. Tell others about your routine. When we advertise our plans, we are more likely to keep them up and keep on living.

V. Prescriptions for Reducing Stress

i. Pamper Yourself

The essentials of pampering oneself must be pleasure-loving, pleasure-seeking and pleasure-creating. Living the life of the senses can lead to better health. Nurture these senses with a long hot bath, a bottle of perfume or a nap in the middle of the day.

Self-pampering is directly related to self-esteem. It is a form of positive reinforcement. You do something good for yourself because you deserve it. Self-pampering implies that you think of yourself with the same respect and caring with which you regard a guest or a loved one. It is a powerful way of asserting your right to happiness, pleasure and good health. Positive reinforcement encourages good behavior and happiness. Pampering yourself is a form of this positive reinforcement.

When you pamper yourself, keep your health in mind. Pampering shouldn't negate all those good things you have done for your good health. If you pamper yourself and it hurts your body, then it is no longer pampering. Positive pampering means choosing things that make you happy and don't hurt your body.

Our prescription: Self-pampering signifies happiness, confidence, satisfaction and good health. Pamper yourself everyday, and live longer.

ii. Laughter Is A Priceless Medicine

> *"Against the assault of laughter, nothing can stand."*
>
> – Mark Twain

> *"The sound of laughter is like the vaulted dome of a temple of happiness."*
>
> – Milan Kundera

Laughter is a natural healer. A hearty laugh is like a spa workout for the muscles of your face, shoulders, diaphragm and abdomen. Your breathing becomes faster and deeper and oxygen floods your bloodstream. Laughter also activates the immune system.

Major hospitals across the nation maintain a "humor cart" of videos, audiotapes and books. The International Center for Humor and Health (1999) is a not-for-profit organization dedicated to spreading the healing art of laughter. They conduct Camp Funnybone for youngsters aged seven to fourteen. The programs help children, many with debilitating or life-threatening diseases, learn how to harness the healing power of laughter.

To burst into laughter, watch a funny sitcom or movie. Try to surround yourself with people who won't bring you down further than you already feel. Do not waste a day. Remember what Sebastian said: "Of all days, the day on which one has not laughed is the one most surely wasted."

Just remember, laughter is a mind relaxer and stress reducer. It triggers the release of endorphins, the chemical in the brain that produces euphoria. It relaxes muscles and reduces perception of pain. It is anti-aging tonic.

Our prescription: Laugh loudly, heartily and frequently.

iii. Prepare For The Unexpected

Life can be full of surprises, small and big, welcome and unwelcome. A child can break her arm in a fall from a bicycle or your son may get involved in a car accident on the way to college. You can run out of gas on a highway or when you come home you find that your air conditioning/ heating system has broken down. An elderly father can fall and break his hip or your apparently healthy spouse suffers a fatal heart attack. Or, you check your numbers and find that you are a winner of a large lottery jackpot. And because surprises come often in all shapes and sizes we must prepare ourselves fully. To face small or big eventualities in life, keep in mind the following ten tips to prepare for unexpected emergencies:

1. Birth of a baby: A happy event, but it can bring several surprises. Ask for help from family members. Keep your doctor's number handy.

2. Birthdays: Buy birthday cards and gifts in bulk and mark birthdays of family members and friends on the calendar.
3. Death: This usually brings heavy burdens if it is unexpected. Collect documents and put them in an easy place to find. The documents should include the will, living will, health and life insurance policies, property deeds, credit cards, bank papers and telephone numbers of friends and family (Fatteh and Fatteh, 1999).
4. House care: In the winter months in cold places many people die from hypothermia. And in summer heat, life can be unbearable without air conditioning. Keep your heating and cooling systems properly maintained.
5. Car care: A breakdown on a highway or even running out of gas can cause major problems especially if you are in the middle of another emergency. Keep it well maintained and refueled.
6. Be prepared to face up to difficult financial times.
7. Carry a cellular phone. Always have on you important telephone numbers of family members, friends, your doctor, etc.
8. When you venture out, carry your identification papers. Leave a note at home indicating where you will be.
9. Medications: Always carry your medications when you leave home. Call your doctor before your run out of your medications.
10. In the case of a major event such as a death in the family seek help and support from friends and family members

Our prescription: Predict and be prepared.

iv. Control Your Anger

When you are angry, your blood pressure rises, you breathe fast and your heart races. Stress hormones are released in high amounts. All these events cause havoc on your immune, cardiovascular and endocrine systems.

A good method of controlling anger is to follow the good old "count to ten" routine. It works. When you are driving along peacefully and someone cuts you off, or your boss screams at you, you get angry. This is when you should start breathing and count to ten. You can also practice square breathing. Count a slow four seconds with each action:

1. Take a deep breath in.
2. Hold it.
3. Exhale.
4. Hold the exhaled breath before taking in another breath.

Try and distract your thoughts with something pleasant. And of course, put it all in perspective. If you are satisfied with yourself, your work and even your driving, then do not let someone else spoil your mood. Keep your mood cheery, it will add years to your life.

v. Learn to Just "Let Go"

"Letting go" can be understood on several different levels. It can mean no longer taking responsibility in every situation or attempting to cause things to happen. For instance, if your child is applying to college, you get deeply involved in every aspect of the process, supervising everything from the essay to the interview. You take a step back and say to yourself, "I will help when needed."

Letting go can also be about relationships. You may feel a responsibility to make a toxic relationship work, when the healthiest move for you could be to walk away. Again. Only you know what's worth letting go and what you should continue to fight for. The point is, not everything is worth the work.

Also, letting go can refer to pain, particularly the pain of losing a loved one through separation or death. No one can tell you when is the appropriate time for you to stop grieving. But when you do, you will feel a palpable sense of relief.

Letting go is often difficult because we feel like we are betraying that person or thing we release ourselves from. Perhaps even harder is the feeling that we are betraying ourselves. Letting go of an attitude or emotion that has been with us for a long time can be very difficult.

Learning to let go means that we have evolved to a new level of consciousness; that we are finally ready to live the life we were meant to live. It is important. Just let go. It can represent the ultimate healing of your spirits. And, it can prepare you for realizing your full potential for health, happiness and long life.

vi. Enjoy The Arts

The arts are a boon for people. They help them develop self-esteem, social interaction, belonging, self-knowledge and self-expression. The whole world is full of arts. Nature is full of them and man has added many. The arts of nature are in the skies, the beauty of the moon and stars, of clouds, sunrises and sunsets. They are in our planet's oceans and landscapes. To the visual joys nature adds the sound of music. There is the gift of music from the ocean waves, winds, and birds. Add to that the pleasures from those in aquariums and zoos.

Man has created many marvels. The art galleries and museums are full of them. The beauty of ballet dancers and voices of opera singers, books and movies, are all there to enjoy. One can spend weeks and months admiring individual efforts of the giants like Picasso and Van Gogh or listen to the musical masterpieces gifted to us by Bach and Mozart. In addition, there are the splendid opera voices of Placido Domingo, Luciano Pavarotti and Andrea Buccelli.

Enjoying arts does not require a special effort. All you need to do is nurture your creative consciousness. Remain open to the joy and essence of experience and to the pleasure and self-knowledge that comes from the exploration of the world.

Just buy yourself a ticket to the ballet or opera. Catch a movie once or twice a month. Browse the Internet. Look up the CD section of your favorite record store. Pick up a new novel. Stop by a local museum or gallery. Or simply admire nature.

The arts intensify life and make it brilliant and beautiful. By embracing the arts in whatever form you choose, you embrace life and make it clearer. Thus, you live longer.

vii. Have Hobbies

Playfulness that makes hobbies is among the psychosocial factors that slows aging and extends life. Play is something we associate with youth. Play releases most painkilling endorphins that make us feel good in mind and body. Hobbies relax us. Hobbies help us find new friends. They preserve our sanity.

You need hobbies at all ages, especially if you are retired. If you are one of those who retired to find you have no outside interests, your first task on the first Monday morning of the rest of your life must be to find a hobby. The idea for this johnny-come-lately to hobbies should be not to challenge yourself but to enjoy. Do not turn play into more stress and tension through an overemphasis on one-on-one competition and achievement. The point of a hobby is that it relieves stress, gives you a break from competition, makes you feel good about yourself and your abilities, and nurtures your creativity. Pick the most enjoyable ones. Here is a list of ten easy-to-pick-up hobbies:

1. Golf, tennis, bowling clubs. You will get exercise and friends.
2. Hiking, biking, skating, skiing groups. They will provide a burst of activity and sociability.
3. Dog, cat and horse shows. They will be fun not only for breeders, but also for trainers, judges and presenters.
4. Coins, stamps, antiques collection. You may be able to turn your hobbies into wise investments.
5. Wine tasting or beer brewing. Or simply fishing.
6. Gourmet cooking club. Start one with friends and neighbors.
7. Social meets. You could join small groups to read poetry, learn a new language, tell jokes, play bridge.
8. Musical instruments. Learn new tunes, new instruments.
9. Traveling, visiting museums and historical sites. Attending sports events. Visiting libraries and bookstores to read and write.
10. Make your home a hobby. Paint, decorate, grow flowers and make it a masterpiece. Living in it will be an added incentive to live longer.

xiii. Enjoy Sex: The Ultimate Stress Buster

On the simplest level, sex is about touch. Human touch makes us feel safe, comfortable and at ease. In fact, physical contact is understood to play such an important role in the human psyche that hospitals are now allowing new mothers to hold their infants as early as possible to establish the mother-baby bond.

But touch is important at any age. In both children and adults, the absence of physical touch is believed to contribute to depression and aggression. As for seniors, when Shere Hite (1981) interviewed thousands of Americans in the 1970s for her acclaimed research, she found that men over sixty considered sex, as one interviewee put it, "the most important thing in life." When career interests and old friends dwindle, she found, people tend to revert to the bases in life, including food and sex.

Sex promotes relaxation more effectively than many medications and alcohol, and relaxation is one of the best stress busters available. Sex also improves physical processes that can indirectly relieve stress. It shields the body from illness, promotes a healthy heart and alleviates many of the symptoms of menopause. It even burns calories, up to 90 an hour!

These advantages come with one caveat, however. When we talk about the stress-relieving effect of sex, we refer to satisfying, safe sex. The definition of satisfying safe sex differs from person to person. Sexual partners who communicate their needs and desires are much more likely to enjoy the full benefit of sex. Be sure to avoid stereotypes, including the old idea that all men require intercourse, while all women are content simply to be held.

In summary, sex reduces stress and promotes sleep. Recognize that sex is for life. That is why George Burns (1983) had this to say: "Sex can be fun after 80, after 90, after 100 and after lunch."

ix. Spot And Stamp Out Stressors

For most of us, some amount of stress in our lives is given. Unfortunately, we tend to put extra stress on ourselves, when we could accomplish the same tasks without it. The main areas in which we are too hard on ourselves are perfectionism, control, people-pleasing and competence. Chapter 19 deals with various aspects of stress. Here is a quick wrap up.

1. Identify stressors at home and deal with them. Don't do it alone. Obtain all the help needed from the family members.
2. Analyze the stresses at work. Seek help from the supervisor and co-workers. Openness is a virtue, use it.
3. Recognize major stress-inducing life events and be prepared to deal with them.
4. Talk to yourself. Find out how you create stresses for yourself. You could be too hard on yourself, sometimes without knowing.
5. Address the problem of worry. It is a major cause of stress.
6. Be armed with stress busters to deal with acute stress.
7. Develop a long-term strategy to deal with chronic stress.
8. Understand how negative stress affects health.
9. Be persistent, eliminate negative thinking and be positive about the outcome of your efforts. Be a believer: stress is beatable.
10. Successfully fielding life's curve balls will help you live healthy and long.

x. Be Contented

> *"Every day is my best day; this is my life; I am not going to have this moment again."*
>
> – Bernie Siegel

"You have the power to make your inner world work for or against you," says psychologist Wayne Dyer (1995): "Use it to create the images of contentment that you want to occur in your material world, and eventually that inner contentment will be the blueprint that you consult as the architect of your everyday life."

The first step to contentment, is being contented with one's self. Believe in yourself. Be thankful for what you are. Do not compare yourself with others. And, do not assess your achievements with reference to others'. Remember what St. Paul said, "I have learned, in whatever state I am, therewith to be content."

To visualize contentment, sit in a quiet room. Close your eyes and take several deep breaths. Let your imagination take over. Imagine all your achievements, imagine all the good things that happened to you. Say this to yourself. This is the only life I have. I am going to enjoy and appreciate it to the fullest. If you are contented, you are more likely to have that life for years to come. The way you should feel is the way Kitty Carlisle Hart said, "Each morning I wake up and say, Dear Lord, I don't want anything better; just send me more of the same."

VI. Prescriptions for Weight Control

i. Prevent Obesity

Let us remind ourselves, obesity is a disease. More importantly it is a preventable disease. This disease is a significant condition that contributes to several other medical problems such as diabetes, high blood pressure, heart failure, high cholesterol and triglycerides, respiratory difficulties, sleep apnea, varicose veins, thrombophlebitis, cancers (of uterus, breast, gallbladder, colon, rectum, and prostate), arthritis, gallstones and fatty liver. Obesity is an exploding epidemic in the Western World. Obesity-related medical problems are second only to tobacco smoking as a leading cause of preventable deaths (JAMA, 1999).

Sedentary life and overeating are major causes of obesity. Inactive life style. Maintaining the right weight at all times must be your ultimate goal. The following ten guidelines will help you to do that:

1. Educate yourself about obesity. Remember if your weight is 20–40% higher than normal, you are mildly obese. If it is 40–99% higher, you are moderately obese, and if it is twice the normal or more, you are severely obese (Rinzler, 1997).
2. Determine the number of calories you should get.
3. Determine the exercise program that will help you burn the number of calories you need to burn off.
4. Eat when you are hungry, stop when you feel full. Regulate eating times.

5. Avoid snacks, junk foods and soft drinks. Drink alcohol in moderation.
6. Do not eat your dinner just before going to bed. Eat only at the dinner table. Do not eat on the run.
7. Maintain a physically active lifestyle at work and at home.
8. Make the weight maintenance commitment lifelong.
9. Prevent obesity in children and adolescents by teaching and showing the above healthy eating habits.
10. Never feel that it is too late to lose weight. You can do it at any time. Go for your goal in small steps.

ii. Obesity: Correct The Cause

The following are important causes of obesity:

1. Overeating is the most common cause of obesity.
2. Sedentary lifestyle is another major factor in causing obesity.
3. Genetic factors.
4. Environmental factors such as poor dietary habits and social stressors can lead to obesity. These are learned behaviors.
5. Medical problems contributing to obesity are underactive thyroid, a hormone disorder called Cushing's Disease, and insulinoma, a condition in which excess insulin production leads to low blood sugars causing one to increase calorie intake to compensate (Harrison, 1994).

As you can see, obesity has multiple causes, but in most cases there is a combination of factors and therefore the approach to obesity management has to be multi-directional. Refer to Chapter 18 for five steps to ensure success in losing weight. Consult your doctor for medical evaluation and treatment options. Work with him and/or a dietitian.

iii. Maintain Optimum Weight

Optimum weight is the same as ideal weight which makes you feel good and keeps you healthy. It also reduces the risk of disease associated with obesity such as heart disease, diabetes, hypertension, arthritis and breathing problems. There are several ways to determine optimum weight.

1. Use the BMI table. If your BMI is between 19 and 25, you have healthy weight. If it is between 25 and 30 you are overweight, and if it is over 30 you are obese. See Appendix B, Table 2.
2. Use the height-weight table (Table 18.1). Get your height in inches and refer to the table and you will get the range of weight in pounds that is good for you.
3. Calculate your weight roughly this way:
Women five feet = 100 lbs, add 5 lbs per extra inch above five feet.
Men five feet = 106 lbs, add 6 lbs per extra inch above five feet.
4. After you determine the ideal weight, if you are 10–20% over it you are overweight. If you are more than 20% over the ideal weight you are obese and if you are 50–100% over the ideal weight, you are morbidly obese.

iv. Count Your Calories: Be A Loser

"To lengthen thy life lessen thy meals."

– Benjamin Franklin

Because our goal is to reach age 100, watching what we eat becomes important. Making sure the foods we eat provide us with the most benefits, calorie counts must become a priority. To do so means keeping track of what we eat, ensuring that we don't take in more calories than we can lose through exercise and other activities.

The first step in watching what you eat should be done with assistance. Consult your doctor and together, establish a healthy diet that you think you can stick with easily. Talk to your doctor about foods you enjoy, and also about healthier ways you can cook your meals.

Another important step in keeping track of your calories is to pay more attention to the things you eat. Foods are required by law to have labels on them, listing the calories, nutritional values and fat content per serving. By reading nutritional labels, you can identify the foods that are good for you.

If you find it difficult to know how many calories you have eaten in a day, try keeping a food diary. Here are ten other ways to keep your calorie intake low:

1. Cut back on your snacks. Junk foods may be empty calories with little to no nutritional value.
2. Find lower-fat alternatives to your favorite foods.
3. If you get the urge for a high-calorie food such as potato chips, pick up an apple as an alternative.
4. If you slip and eat unhealthy food, don't be too hard on yourself. Compensate for it later in the day or the next day.
5. Cut down on empty calorie foods and drinks, such as soft drinks.
6. If you get the urge to eat, try to distract yourself with another engaging activity.
7. Keep track of your food intake, and use it as a motivational tool. Keep a food diary.
8. Consult your doctor on what kinds of food you should be eating.
9. Read books to help you shape a diet plan that works for you.
10. Remember that counting your calories is for your health.

Our prescription: Count calories and make food your medicine.

v. Exercise For Weight Loss

Here are some important facts:

1. Weight gain occurs when energy or caloric intake is greater than energy expenditure. Exercise is one of the most beneficial ways to lose weight.
2. Exercise is a great way to burn calories and burning calories allows you to lose weight.
3. There are many different forms of exercise and each one provides a different amount of calorie loss. Table 11.1 shows the calorie loss for different exercises.
4. Building up your exercise regimen slowly is advisable, if you are just starting a work out program.

100 Prescriptions to Live to be 100

5. If you are an established exerciser, and want to lose more weight, it is necessary for you to do exercises that burn more calories.
6. Remember that you still have to watch what you eat. Exercising does not give you free license to have that extra piece of cake.
7. Aging does alter your metabolism. Exercise among the elderly is important and is still an effective means of weight loss.
8. If you are not consistent in exercising, it is possible that you will rebound and put on weight again.
9. If you are obese, you may have difficulty doing strenuous activities because of joint pain or weakness or difficulty breathing. Use exercises which do not need as much weight bearing or rough physical activity such as swimming and slow walking.
10. It does take time for the body to get to the point where fat stores are used for calories. That is why exercise does not lead to weight loss overnight. Do not get on the scale one day after exercising and be discouraged by seeing no change. It takes time, persistence and patience.

vi. Seek Behavior Modification Counseling

Behavior modification is a powerful tool for people looking to lose weight. It should consist of planning, record-keeping, creating menus, and creating and sticking with an exercise program. Additionally, emotional support is provided via group therapy or individual counseling. Why should you seek behavior modification counseling? Here are ten reasons:

1. It offers a normal, natural way to lose weight.
2. You learn from a trained professional how to change your lifestyle in order to lose weight.
3. There are support groups with other patients who are going through the same problems you are experiencing. It allows for the realization that you are not alone.
4. You learn how to take care of yourself, rather than be dependent on drugs or "miracle cures."
5. A gradual pace allows you time to adjust to the changes.

6. You get a comparative sense of your success.
7. You learn to control your urges and eat right.
8. You develop a mindset that makes it more difficult for you to "slip" back into old habits.
9. It teaches you new ways to eat and eat healthy.
10. It emphasizes the importance of the nuts and bolts of weight maintenance.

Your prescription: Behave yourself. With the power of your mind, empower your body.

vii. Snack Sensibly

At any given time, 25% of men and 45% of women are actively trying to lose weight. That means millions of people are swearing off potato chips and ice cream or wish they could. Remember, snacks are a treat, not a food group. They are for suppressing your appetite for main meals, not for filling up between meals.

If you have to snack, simply make some small modifications in your diet. Be creative. Substitute delicious nonfat frozen yogurt for ice cream. Use low fat plain yogurt instead of sour cream in dips, dressings or spreads. Spread reduced fat cheeses on melba toast instead of whole milk cheeses on crackers. And become a supermarket detective, scanning nutrition labels for words such as low, light, or reduced. Just beware, low fat doesn't always mean low calorie, and it's calories that pack on the pounds.

Snacks beat hunger and stop you from overeating at mealtime. Busy people on the go, take a look at these healthy snacks.

1. Whole-grain cereal with skim milk and berries.
2. Low fat granola bar and canned pineapple.
3. Gingersnaps with skim or low fat milk.
4. Light microwave popcorn.
5. Whole-grain crackers and cottage cheese.
6. Non-fat yogurt and Fig Newtons.

TABLE 25.3
Calories in Soda

Soda	Serving Size	Calories	Sodium	Carb
Coke	8 oz	97	9	27
Pepsi	8 oz	105	2	27
Sprite	8 oz	100	30	26
Dr. Pepper	8 oz	130	55	40
Mountain Dew	8 oz	118	21	30
Sunkist	8 oz	140	45	35
Diet Coke	8 oz	1	4	trace
Diet Pepsi	8 oz	1	trace	trace
Canada Dry Ginger Ale	8 oz	90	15	24

7. Bagel with peanut butter and fruit.
8. Vanilla wafers and fruit.
9. A portion of leftovers from your healthy lunch for a mid-afternoon snack.
10. A juicy apple and a slice of low fat cheese.

Our prescription: Eat healthy snacks to suppress your appetite for main meals, and not for filling up between meals.

viii. Limit Your Soft Drinks

There are a number of different soft drinks, regular and diet, caffeinated and not, sugared and sugar-free. Table 25.3 shows the calorie and salt amounts in some of them (Natow and Hestin, 1999). Soft drinks taste good. That is because of the high sugar and salt content.

To cut calories, salt and sugar, limit the soft drinks. The best way to limit your soft drinks is to find an alternative drink that you find to be tasty. Good alternatives are frozen fruit drink, lemon iced tea or even water with a slice of lemon or lime.

Caffeine is another element found in soft drinks. While it may be all right to have some caffeine during the day, it is not a good idea to have too much at night. This will keep you up longer.

ix. Use Diet Pills Only Under Medical Supervision

The use of diet pills is rampant. Many patients tend to self treat their weight problem with prescribed medications and over-the-counter products. Non-compliance with the proper use of prescribed drugs can create health hazards. (Note the side effects of diet pills in Table 18.3.) Overdose or improper use can be disastrous. Non-prescription drugs can be particularly dangerous because their composition is not always defined or controlled. Use any kind of diet pill only with your physician's approval and under strict medical supervision. Complete compliance with your physician's advice will keep you safer.

x. Don't Be A Yo-Yo: Be Consistent

In our medical practice we have hundreds of patients enrolled for weight loss and weight maintenance programs. The patients are advised at the outset that losing weight will be easy but maintaining the weight will be difficult and will require constant efforts. They are started with psychological counseling and are urged to lose weight slowly. For weight loss we prescribe an appetite suppressant. With this, the diet advice requires eating a good breakfast, moderate sized lunch and dinner adding up to 1200 to 1500 calories. It is stressed that snacks, soft drinks and desserts be eliminated. An exercise program suitable to the patient is discussed. The program is extremely successful as far as weight loss is concerned; almost all of the patients lose weight. However, the sad part of the story is that the patients become non-compliant during the weight maintenance phase and most fail to keep the appointments. Another disappointing aspect of the program is that many regain the weight and about half of all dropouts come back to rejoin the program, some more than once. Those are the ones who belong to the "yo-yo" category.

The "yo-yo" problem is also called weight cycling—the phenomenon of repeatedly losing and regaining weight. The people going through weight cycling have lack of determination and discipline, poor self esteem and eating disorders. They develop a slower metabolic rate; gain weight with fewer calories and their weight management becomes more difficult. Their confidence wanes.

The cycle of "weight gain, weight loss, weight gain" is psychologically devastating and defeating to patients. Their resolve to solve the problem weakens. The real prescription for sustained weight loss must include the following:

1. Avoid quick-fix diets.
2. Avoid weight loss gimmicks.
3. Avoid medical offices where pills are dished out without proper medical examination, laboratory tests and EKG and where the physician does not see you.
4. Be committed to total compliance during weight loss phase as well as weight maintenance phase.
5. Be determined and disciplined.
6. Opt for slow long-term method rather than short-term results.
7. Make gradual and lasting changes in your eating habits.
8. Avoid snacking, sodas and desserts.
9. Go for positive reinforcement sessions.
10. Exercise regularly.

Your prescription: Complete dedication to weight maintenance resolution is the way to a healthy and longer life. If you have two wardrobes, get rid of the "fat" one and keep the "skinny" one forever.

VII. Social, Emotional Prescriptions

i. Don't Be a Loner: Be a People Person

"Art thou lonely, O my brother? Share thy little with another! Stretch a hand to one unfriended, and the loneliness is ended."
– William Arthur Dunkerly

"Loneliness and the feeling of being unwanted is the most terrible poverty."
– Mother Teresa. (Gonzalez-Balado, 1996)

A 26-year-old man with no siblings, a woman age 40, whose husband was recently killed in a car accident, and a 72 year old man whose siblings and parents were killed in World War II, came to us for psychological counseling. The principal complaint of each was loneliness.

No matter what the cause of loneliness is, the state of being lonely itself, promotes illness and suffering. Friendship heals and loneliness kills. Loneliness and isolation lead to depression. A person who is lonely is likely to eat more, exercise less, abuse drugs, drink alcohol, and smoke. The above three patients admitted to doing all these things. Depression induced by loneliness and alienation can lead to suicides. We have seen many suicide notes citing loneliness as a reason to commit suicide.

To fight off loneliness there are many things one can do. Some concern others, many concern you. As for others, it is important to do and say things that would attract them to you. Remember these ten things:

1. Regard others as more important than yourself.
2. Demonstrate concern and sensitivity for others.
3. Listen to them, appreciate them and encourage them.
4. Don't demean them or undermine them.
5. Appreciate them and forgive them. This is the way to win them.
6. When you talk, put yourself in someone else's place. Say nice things. Heed Bahn's advice, "Speak kind words and you will hear kind echoes."

7. Be generous to others.
8. Extend a helping hand to others whenever you can.
9. Demonstrate love and affection.
10. Never decline an invitation to a party, dinner or any other social activity and practice all of the above when you are with others.

In the battle to beat loneliness there are ten things you can do:

1. Be confident and leader-like.
2. Maintain a healthy emotional state.
3. Don't be oversensitive or moody.
4. Put aside pride and negativism.
5. Don't be critical or boastful.
6. Don't hibernate, be social.
7. Live with loved ones, have close friends.
8. Don't be weak, dependent and helpless.
9. Participate in group activities.
10. Stay involved with people.

Our prescription: Remember that the people who are not lonely live longer. Be a people person.

ii. Live With Loved Ones

"If you don't have the support and love and caring and concern that you get from a family, you don't have much at all."

– Morrie Schwartz in Tuesdays with Morrie by Mitch Albom (1997)

It hurts when a marriage fails and you get separated. This creates loneliness, insecurity, sadness and depression. Divorce brings similar maladies. The spirit of interdependence breaks, the bonds of love disappear and the joys of physical togetherness get shattered. This is why it is so important to make a few sacrifices, preserve your marriage and family. Love and live with that one individual you vowed to share your life with.

The bonuses of a marriage are children and grandchildren. They become an automatic part of your life adding to the priceless elements of life's pleasures. Just being around the hustle and bustle of children and grandchildren will keep you feeling young.

Human beings need to be needed. Don't look for nursing homes or retirement homes for your parents and grandparents. Keeping them with you will help them live longer and you happier. On the most basic level, if there is a medical emergency, day or night, you will be by their side to call an ambulance, drive them to a hospital or render care at home. If you are old and sick needing constant care, living with loved ones is especially critical for you.

In summary, if you are a member of a household, chances are good that in the course of a day, you will be called upon to open a jar, tie a shoelace, fill in a cross word puzzle clue or otherwise help another human being. The next time your spouse or granddaughter makes one of these simple requests of you, be grateful. They are among the most effective of all prescriptions for long life.

iii. Maintain A Happy Marriage/Relationship

Good marriages and relationships can make for a good long life. This is because intimacy in relationships expands our souls, cements the bond, creates independence, and results in the ultimate happiness. Both partners must understand that there are some basic components that formulates a good marriage or relationship. They require both partners to strive to be good friends, respect each other and be generous to each other. They must develop a common set of good values and thrive on them together. True caring calls for making sacrifices and true harmony demands compromises. Also, forgiving and asking for forgiveness are potent cementing forces. While keeping in mind all these elements in a happy marriage or relationship, remember that little things make a big difference. Here are ten important tips:

1. Communicate fully, openly and kindly. Talk to your spouse for at least five minutes face-to-face every day. Maintain eye contact at all times.

2. Go for honeymoons, often. Plan trips together. Pick the places and activities both can share and enjoy.
3. Surprise your spouse with a mystery trip, a gift or simply a love note (Bradshaw, 1992).
4. Give compliments. Appreciate your spouse's clothes or appearance. Say nice things about the work done by your spouse.
5. Agree to disagree but disagree respectfully with rational, logical discussion. Be open and do not leave the issues unresolved.
6. Share chores. Eat together. Walk, swim or bicycle together.
7. Have some interests suited to each partner.
8. Share interests, responsibilities and experiences. Attend children's school and sports activities together.
9. Be polite always to each other.
10. Do not take your spouse for granted. Do not forget wedding anniversary dates, father's/mother's days and birthdays. A gift, flowers and a candle light dinner will express a lot.

A right prescription for maintaining a happy marriage or relationship must include the elements of giving, forgiving, compromising, sacrificing, respecting, and loving.

iv. Make And Keep Close Friends

"And let your best be your friend. If he must know the ebb of your tide, let him know its flood also. For what is your friend that you should seek him with hours to kill? Seek him always with hours to live."

– Khalil Gibran

True friendship is a two way traffic. Each side cares and each side benefits. Serving as an emotional support, your friend is as important to your health and well-being as receiving that support, To be needed, and to be able to provide that need, keeps us feeling good about ourselves. And that's what gets us up everyday for more.

For emotional support, for times of emergencies and for day-to-day, heart-to-heart communications we need true friends. These are the people who care for you and you care for them. Friends are the people you feel like talking to everyday. They share your excitement, they reduce your pain and relieve your stress.

If you have close friends, you will never feel lonely or isolated. You will enhance happiness, you will be more confident and emotionally upbeat.

v. Express Feelings Fully

Everyone has feelings. Some express, some don't. To be truly alive is to feel and to express feelings. That is one of the joys and responsibilities of living. Pent-up emotions don't just disappear; they fester and do us harm. People who hold things in create built-in stress. Here are ten benefits of expressing feelings fully:

1. You maintain a clean relationship.
2. You eliminate uneasiness in the relationship.
3. You get certified as open and straight forward.
4. You let your rights be known.
5. You put the other person at ease.
6. You remove doubts and confusion.
7. You strengthen the relationship.
8. You reduce stress, stomach aches and other problems for yourself.
9. You reduce stress, stomach aches and other problems for your spouse or friend.
10. You live longer.

vi. Participate In Group Activities, Senior Olympics

Group activities take you outside of yourself. They require negotiation and compromise, cooperation and team spirit. They get you laughing or yelling. They always leave you feeling good. If you live alone and don't know that many people, try some of these ten ways to join a group (AARP, 1987).

1. Find a house of worship that suits your religious affiliation and personal preference.
2. If you are a parent of young children, join your PTA.

3. Participate in or organize a Neighborhood Watch.
4. Join a photography, stamp collection or other club that shares your interests.
5. Join an athletic league for bowling, tennis, etc.
6. Take a class at an adult education program or college.
7. Sign up for a guided tour.
8. Join a support group for an illness or personal challenge.
9. Volunteer in a formalized program.
10. Join a professional organization even if you are retired.

vii. Be Generous: Help, Volunteer

"We make a living by what we get, but we make a life by what we give."

– Norman McEvan

People who need people may be the luckiest people in the world, but people who help people are among the healthiest. A little volunteer work fetches a bonus. Seniors who volunteer just an hour a day tend to live longer than those who do not.

Samuel Johnson said "Always set a high value on spontaneous kindness." You feel good when you help. Remember what John Andrew Holmes said "There is no experience better for the heart than reaching down and lifting someone up." Serving others gets us thinking about something other than our own problems. It gets us moving and we experience good feelings. Here are ten ways to serve others:

1. Visit a sick friend
2. Help at your house of worship, to keep it well maintained.
3. Speak up for a good cause; distribute flyers for a good purpose.
4. Volunteer at a hospital "Real generosity is doing something nice for someone who'll never find it out." - Frank A. Clark
5. Offer to do chores for an elderly neighbor.
6. Invite someone who lives alone to share a meal.
7. On your way to the store ask a neighbor if you can pick up something for him or her.

8. Volunteer at a senior center, retirement home, nursing home or hospice.
9. Serve at a soup kitchen for the homeless.
10. Offer to baby-sit for a friend.

Your prescription: (from Madelina S. Bridges) "Give to the world the best you have, and the best will come back to you."

viii. Dance Into The 21st Century

Dancing is an aerobic exercise with all the benefits that regular exercise can provide, such as improved cardiovascular activity, weight loss and a stronger heart. Not only is dancing a popular form of exercising, it's also a wonderful form of socializing. Many local community centers and senior centers offer senior dance classes, with the styles ranging from ballroom dancing to country line dancing. It can be a great way to meet people outside of your community and make new friends. Here are ten reasons to go dancing:

1. Health benefits of dancing are as good as those of other aerobic exercises if you keep moving at a steady pace.
2. It requires no special equipment or training.
3. Finding a place to dance is easy. Many clubs, restaurants, community centers, senior centers, churches and synagogues offer social dances and dance classes.
4. You make more friends. Social dancing is an especially good way to meet people since you change partners often and because there are many people who attend from different walks of life.
5. Dancing is something you can do at home with your child or spouse, or out with a group of friends.
6. Getting out of the house is a good way to combat loneliness since you can't dance alone.
7. There is a kind of dancing to suit almost any taste and attitude.
8. You can lose weight from dancing since it is an exercise. You can burn up to 500 calories per hour doing aerobic dancing.

9. Anyone can dance, at any age.
10. Most importantly, dancing is a relaxing exercise and clean fun, good for the body, mind and longevity.

Our prescription: Dancing is a fun and easy exercise that is good for your body. Try it! Do it once a week. It all adds up to more years of active life.

ix. Practice Safe Sex

There is no such thing as 100% safe sex, at any age. Any behavior involving the exchange of body fluids is a potential health risk. That may explain why sexually transmitted diseases (STDs) including genital herpes, gonorrhea, syphilis and AIDS are among the most common contagious diseases, affecting one in four Americans, with 12 million new cases each year. Heterosexual sex is the world's fastest growing transmitter of HIV. Everyone who has had unsafe sex in the past decade is at risk.

You can protect yourself against STDs by practicing "safer sex." Make sure that a prospective sexual partner is not infected with HIV. He or she must have had two negative HIV antibody tests, six months apart from the time of their last possible exposure.

Latex condoms, when used correctly and consistently, can prevent the exchange of body fluids during intercourse. Be sure to have a spare in case one of them has a hole or is otherwise defective.

Communication is another winning strategy. Know who you're sleeping with. Bring up the topic of safer sex before you have a few drinks and long before you reach the bedroom. Get tested together. And always practice the three R's: respect, responsibility and the right to say "no". Remember the following are unsafe practices with high risk of sexually transmitted diseases including HIV infection:

1. Vaginal intercourse without a condom with an infected individual.
2. Oral—anal contact.
3. Anal sex with an infected partner without protection.

4. Anal douching with anal sex.
5. Multiple sex partners.
6. Oral sex.

On the other hand, the following are safe practices:

1. Sexual abstinence.
2. Monogamous sexual relations between uninfected partners.
3. Self masturbation and masturbation of partner with no broken skin.
4. Hugging, touching, stroking.
5. Dry kissing.

x. Travel: Expand Your Mind

To open your mind to new activities, languages, historical sites and foods—travel. On travels you meet people. You exercise your mind and body. And if all those postcards are true, you have a wonderful time. You can visit friends or relatives across the state, across a country.

If you really want to expand your mind when you travel, pick up a comprehensive guidebook and get to know the history, culture, geography, and even the language of your destination. You can participate in educational courses in the arts and sciences of a new culture in your own hometowns or around the world.

However you choose to travel, bear in mind the following ways to get the most out of your adventure (Peterson, 1997):

1. Travel with patience. Understand that other cultures operate on different standards.. Learn from them. See a new side to things.
2. Don't be in a rush. Take time and enjoy the sites and people.
3. Travel with expectations of positive reward. Have a positive attitude and you will enjoy more.
4. Travel hopefully. Most plans work out if you think they will.
5. Travel humbly, and your hosts will appreciate you.
6. Travel courteously. Be considerate of the people in the country you are visiting. Follow them. Be polite, respectful and cheerful.
7. Travel with an open mind. You will learn many new things.
8. Travel with curiosity. It's the best way to learn.

9. Travel with imagination. It makes every experience fun and more enlightening. Travel adventurously. Try new places, new foods, new activities.
10. Travel with a relaxed mind.

Finally, whenever possible, travel with a friend or family. Sharing life's pleasures is a wonderful way to keep yourself healthy and happy.

VIII. Mental – Spiritual Prescriptions

i. Think Young, Associate with the Young

> *"For age is opportunity no less than youth itself, though in another dress."*
>
> – Longfellow

The best way to feel young is to play with your children and grandchildren! Children experience the world as a wondrous, awe-inspiring place. If you want to recapture the sense of excitement at waking up every morning, be with children. They say and do the darnest things. Their actions and words are youth-promoting elixirs. Their questions will reflect spirituality; their statements will teach you honesty. Their movements will show purpose and their benign smiles and laughter will fill the air with ecstatic joy.

Younger people will give you an altered sense of yourself. You will act young, and think young, as they do. Overall, you will become more active spiritually, mentally and physically. You will be healthier and live longer.

ii. Develop A Will To Enjoy Life

Among the factors that extend longevity and slow the aging process are: job satisfaction, a happy marriage, the ability to laugh easily, taking at least one week's vacation every year and feelings of personal happiness. Not coincidentally, each of these factors influences whether, and how we enjoy life.

Learn how to enjoy life. Overcome the obstacles that prevent you from living the life you want.

1. Look out for yourself.
2. Do what is important for yourself.
3. Ease up on your commitments.
4. Place less importance on money than is necessary.
5. Enjoy the pleasures of being part of a group.
6. Protect your spiritual well being.

iii. Say A Nice Thing To Someone Everyday

"Speak kind words and you will hear kind echoes."
– Bahn

"People don't care how much you know until they know how much you care."
– John Maxwell

To be worthy of longevity, we must be truly human. Worthy of longevity! What a concept! By taking longevity onto a higher moral plane, each of us can extend our life span by being a good person who deserves to be alive a little longer. And given that we are social creatures in a complex world, doesn't it make sense that people who make life a little better or easier for others would earn that right?

We can also think of being nice to people on a nuts-and-bolts level, of course. We know that those at greatest risk of heart disease tend toward cynicism, anger and aggression. So it follows that making a conscious effort to be nice would tend to deflect those heart-hurtful tendencies. Wayne Dyer (1999) puts it still another way: "Practice being kind instead of being right."

Saying something nice to someone every day can bring you extra days of life. Here are ten simple ways to say something nice:

1. Compliment a co-worker on his or her appearance. Ask about a boss or coworker's family.
2. Recognize a waiter or flight attendant for a job well done.

3. Tell someone you haven't met in a long time how glad you are to see him or her again.
4. When you get a phone call, mention how nice it is to hear the person's voice.
5. Say "please" and "thank you" when it's not expected.
6. Tell your spouse, family member or friend that you care about her or him.
7. Do a simple favor, such as opening a car door.
8. Tell a friend you'd like to spend more time with him or her.
9. Say anything good to someone you usually ignore.
10. Say caring words.

iv. Develop Personal Independence

Personal independence is a cause for celebration. Dependence on others prevents us from achieving personal growth and happiness. A mark of personal independence is trusting your intuition, and doing things for yourself. Here is an easy way to learn how: Make a decision. Then see if you can live with it. You can enjoy personal independence in many ways. Here are ten ways to enjoy personal independence:

1. By learning to say "no".
2. By choosing to do what you feel you should do, and reducing unwanted commitments.
3. By putting yourself as number one.
4. By wearing what you feel is appropriate.
5. By choosing the place you want to live in.
6. By working at a job of your choice.
7. By "marching to your own drummer" and being emotionally confident.
8. By hanging onto relationships good for you and dropping the rest.
9. By owning things you do not have to share.
10. By just being you.

Nurture independence. Your life will be happier and healthier.

v. Pray: Ten Proven Parameters

> *"I pray Thee, O God, that I may be beautiful again."*
>
> – Socrates

Norman Vincent Peale once said: "One of the greatest of all efficiency methods is a pray power." Here are ten powers of praying:

1. Prayer promotes health and longevity. Church-goers are known to smoke less, are less likely to abuse alcohol than non church-goers and hence are healthier and live longer. In a comprehensive review of all the scientific literature on healing and spirituality, Matthews and his associates (1994) identified the profound influence of religious factors on health and longevity. The greater a person's religious commitment, they found, the better his or her overall health and the longer his or her survival.
2. Prayer accelerates healing. A study from Northwestern University Medical School in 1990 showed that after hip surgery the women with strong religious faith got on their feet faster than non-believers.
3. Praying reduces stress by lowering the levels of the stress hormone, cortisol.
4. Prayer is a good medicine for the mind and the body. It calms the mind and promotes peace. It reduces blood pressure, slows the heart rate and lowers the respiratory rate (Dossey, 1996).
5. Prayer strengthens the immune system. A study in 1988 from the Randolph Byrd University of California in San Francisco proved this: The patients singled out for prayer required fewer antibiotics, suffered less congestive heart failure and were more able to fight off pneumonia.
6. Praying lowers death rates. This is a conclusion derived from the California Public Health Foundation (Myers, 2000). The researchers studied 5,000 people for 28 years. They demonstrated that persons who regularly attended religious services showed death rates 65% less than those who rarely attended religious services.

7. Prayer helps survival after surgery. A study from the Dartmouth–Hitchcock Medical Center concluded that heart patients deriving comfort from religious beliefs were three times more likely to survive bypass surgery than those of little faith.
8. Prayer also helps recovery. The heart patients with strong friend and family support and deep religious convictions are 14 times more likely to recover than those with few friends and little faith in religion.
9. Where there is prayer, there is joy, peace and love, all elements contributing to health.
10. Praying is an avenue to fellowship, to purity, to contentment and to discipline, all major factors enhancing longevity.

Praying allows our minds to leave behind the polluting thoughts and pressures of our workday world, and allows us to experience a purer, healthier existence. So take time off for a regular vacation from the world through prayers.

vi. Meditate

Meditation is a mental exercise in which the mind, in a state of relaxed awareness focuses on a word, object or an image. This allows one's thoughts to be freed from the involvement in the day-to-day stresses and distractions. It can also be described as a state of relaxed passive attention to a repetitive, absorbing stimulus that turns off the "inner dialogue" or turmoil. The practice of meditation results in several beneficial effects:

1. Meditation helps retrieve deeper thoughts and feelings and creates spiritual awareness.
2. Deep restfulness achieved by meditation strengthens the mind. It quiets the mind and makes you experience an inner sense of peace, happiness and well being.
3. It improves concentration.
4. It lowers blood pressure, heart rate, respiratory rate and oxygen consumption.

5. It helps you endure pain better.
6. Meditation helps you listen to yourself and promotes reassurance and confidence.
7. Meditation gives you added power from the ability to focus without distraction, and allows you to enjoy your senses more fully.
8. It is known to enhance immune functions.
9. It rejuvenates you and gives you a fresh start.
10. Meditation reduces stress by diminishing tissue sensitivity to stress hormones and helps you to live better and longer.

Meditate to get closer to your soul. Here is how to do it:

1. Fix regular times for meditation exercise. Select a place with the least noise or other distractions.
2. Sit on a comfortable floor with a natural posture. Close your eyelids with your eyes turned slightly inwards but without strain.
3. Breathe in slowly, steadily and fully, and concurrently raise your shoulders.
4. Exhale slowly, steadily and fully, and concurrently lower your shoulders.
5. Repeat inhalation/exhalation exercise several times, and stay in a quiet state of mind for five or more minutes.
6. Relax every muscle of the body consciously by adopting the most comfortable posture.
7. Repeat muscle relaxation procedure several times, and stay quiet for five minutes or longer.
8. Concentrate on a word (e.g. om, shalom, amen, salaam, Allah) or mantra and repeat it or concentrate on an object to lead the mind out of the thinking process, and into mental silence.
9. Stay in a quiet state of mind, thoroughly relaxed for a few minutes.
10. Meditate for 15–30 minutes every day and enjoy a pleasant experience of complete absorption.

Final words: Cost free, effective stress reducer and health promoter. It will add many extra days to your life.

vii. Love

> *" A new commandment I give to you, that you love one another"*
>
> – Jesus

> *"Love comes from God, and everyone who loves is begotten by God and knows God; those who don't love don't know God, for God is love."*
>
> – I John 4:7

"As long as we love," notes Leo Buscaglia (1992), "we remain young. Love is the long-sought Fountain of Youth." That's because love is a commitment. It is a reaching out of ourselves to embrace another person, not only physically but also mentally, emotionally and spiritually.

Love is contagious. Love generates joy. The joy of loving emanates from talking, sharing, laughing, giving, and even grieving. When we love, we open ourselves up to a host of related emotions and experiences, from expressing our deepest thoughts and feelings to involving ourselves with our loved ones. When we love, we learn. We know others. We find out what they like or dislike. We know how they love. We learn to double our love. Fruit of service to others is love.

When you experience the job that comes with loving and being loved, your brain releases "pleasure" chemicals called endorphins, which help reduce pain and fatigue, and ease stress. Love is a tonic we can self-prescribe. Look for love and you will find it. Remember Victor Hugo's words: "The supreme happiness of life is the conviction that we are loved." Love, you may not be aware, just is: give it.

viii. Seek Peace

Peace is a sense of emotional and spiritual well-being. If we experience it in our hearts, we will share it with others. Peace comes when we mentally, emotionally, spiritually and sometimes physically disconnect ourselves from conflicts and responsibilities.

Peace brings relief from stress. There are a number of techniques for achieving peace, such as hypnotic suggestion, prayer, yoga and medication, and guided imagery. In our modern world, the journey to inner peace may mean that we are not always available via phones and faxes, e-mails, and snail mails that pile up on our desks and in our lives. We must learn to let all of that go for a while. This will create an immensely freeing feeling and with it peace.

When we attain peace it helps us reset priorities and it encourages us to think beyond the here-and-now and onto a higher plane. Once we experience it on a regular basis, the joys of life mount. Just be ready for the journey to peace, never look back. This will improve your odds of living longer.

ix. Celebrate Each Day Of Life

Each new day is a milestone. You've been given another opportunity to enjoy life. Isn't that cause for celebration? Celebrate with loved ones. Celebrate with good thoughts and generous acts. Celebrate by caring for your life. Life is a precious gift from the hand of God. Strive to make the most of it. Here are ten ways to celebrate each day of your life:

1. Express your feeling of love to those closest to you.
2. Give yourself a gift.
3. Experience nature.
4. Do someone a favor; extend a helping hand.
5. Nurture yourself with good food and exercise.
6. Practice relaxation.
7. Exercise your spiritual potential.
8. Indulge your senses with pleasurable food and drink.
9. Enjoy the arts.
10. Create something that gives you pleasure.

All this done every day with a positive attitude will give you extra seconds, minutes or even hours and when these bonuses are added up you will have not just a long, long life but a happy one.

x. Be Resilient

Two people can start out life with an impoverished, alcoholic father and overburdened mother. One can become a criminal, while the other can grow up to become Frank McCourt, author of the Pulitzer Prize-winning memoir *Angela's Ashes* (Brody, 1997, p. 391). The difference is resilience. Here are famous examples of resilience:

1. Soap queen Susan Lucci was nominated for more Emmys than she can count on both hands. Each year she held her head high and joked about the awards process, but she did not give up. Her resilience paid off. Finally she won in 1999.
2. Robert Pirsig's *Zen and the Art of Motorcycle Maintenance* was rejected by dozens of publishers. He persisted and it became a big bestseller.
3. Actor Christopher Reeve was paralyzed from the neck down after a riding accident but fought back all his physical adversities to star in and direct movies.
4. Theoretical physicist Stephen Hawking, Ph.D., overcame Lou Gehrig's disease to become one of our most esteemed scientists.
5. Skater Nancy Kerrigan was seriously injured before competing in the Winter Olympics, but rebounded to win a silver medal.
6. Indian Prime Minister Indira Gandhi and Pakistani Prime Minister Benazir Bhutto were swept out of office but returned to power with their persistence.
7. South African President Nelson Mandela was jailed for over a quarter of a century before becoming a international hero and Nobel Prize winner.
8. National Hockey League referee Paul Stewart beat cancer to return to the game and set up a national cancer foundation.
9. Veteran actress Tuesday Weld was a child alcoholic who went on to become a major movie star.
10. Football quarterback Doug Flutie established a foundation for autism after his son was diagnosed with the disorder.

Our prescription: As you can see, you can't keep a strong person down. Be resilient and come out ahead.

IX. Good General Prescriptions

i. Beat Burnout

> *"Choose a job you love and you will never have to work."*
>
> – Confucius

The term "burnout" is commonly used to describe emotional exhaustion, cynicism and negative stress. Burnout at work is slightly complicated. "It is likely to occur when we invest too much of ourselves in the job," explains Paul Stevens (1995) founder of the Center for Worklife counseling. "Burnout diminishes our feelings of being worthwhile."

Burnout can occur in any profession, at any time. It can affect any worker who must hide displeasure, who no longer cares about the job, or who no longer feels comfortable in the work environment. Characterized by frustration, irritability, and loss of energy it reveals itself as low achievement, increased errors and isolation.

Burnout can lead to health-hazardous behaviors such as drug abuse, drinking to excess, or overeating and it contributes to depression, high blood pressure, heart attack, a compromised immune system, ulcers, and even cancer. The first step to fighting burnout is regular exercise, a healthy diet, and plenty of rest. Next, do what you can to relieve on-the-job tension. In many cases, the third step is out the door.

Our prescription: Don't get burned with a burnout.

ii. Learn To Cope

Coping means exchanging a bad mood for good and trading pain for contentment. Coping well transforms negative beliefs, establishes healthy relationships, helps express your full range of emotions, and perhaps most importantly, nurtures yourself.

Coping skills come in three types: relaxation techniques such as meditation and progressive muscle relaxation, mental techniques such as visualization and guided imagery and situational techniques, including humor, social support and assertiveness. The key to using these coping skills is to match the technique to the problem. To this end, follow the Ornstein and Sobel technique (1996). If the problem is important and changeable use imagery, assertiveness, social support, or planning and goal setting. If it is important and unchangeable, try to recast the way you think and feel about the problem. Or, see if a small part of the problem is changeable, and work on that. If this doesn't work try to distract yourself, help others, seek social support, nurture your senses, use relaxation, imagery, humor or exercise.

If it is unimportant and changeable, let the problem go. If it is unimportant and unchangeable, ignore the problem. If you can't, try relaxation, imagery, humor and distractions. To cope successfully keep physically fit, get enough rest, make life simple, reduce stress, get involved, pace yourself, focus on positives, learn to say "no", laugh, get enough sleep, relax, and depend on a support system (Johnson and Klein, 1994).

iii. Learn to Develop Self-Respect

Self respect connects your mind to your body. It improves your mental attitude and builds mental strength. These characteristics strengthen the body, offering it a greater sense of survival.

Self respect brings reassurance and peace. You will socialize better and make more friends. You will compete more vigorously. You will perform better at work and you will be happier at home. Self respect, brings health benefits. It lowers stress level, and strengthens immune system. The best prescription you can create for yourself; Develop, and maintain respect for yourself.

iv. Believe in Yourself and Your Power to Heal

Personal power is within us and all of us can utilize it. To do this we must discard negative thinking and believe that all odds are in our favor. This builds that power. We must believe in ourselves. Only when we believe in our power to heal ourselves can we improve our destiny. The power within us can accelerate recovery from illnesses. The improved confidence betters us to deal with our health problems. This is a way to increase longevity.

v. Sustain A Positive Attitude

"It is no secret, the people who live long are those who long to live."

– Anonymous

"Success is ninety-nine percent mental attitude."

– Rosseau

Keeping your chin up may be the single most important thing you can do to achieve longevity, and more importantly, to enjoy the extra years you earn. The better you feel about yourself and your life, the more incentive you have to be healthy and strive to reach the century mark. Consider the following points:

1. When you're feeling down, compare yourself to that positive person you imagined. Become that person. *"Your world is as big as you make it."* – George Douglas Johnson.
2. A positive attitude can make a difference between success and failure. Negativism will keep you from enjoying life. Live one day at a time positively, and live fully. George Burns had this to say: *"There is nothing more important than a positive attitude, I think."*
3. A positive attitude keeps your mind alert and more capable of dealing with stress.
4. A positive attitude helps create mental, emotional, physical and spiritual good health.
5. A positive attitude helps avoid harmful behavior like drinking excessively, smoking and allowing dark thoughts to overwhelm you.

Our prescription: Make your body language reflect positive attitude. Fake it 'til you make it. Put on a smile, and get out of the house. Listen to Virginia Woolf: "Arrange whatever pieces come your way." And, don't forget what C.W. Longenecker said: "Life's battles don't always go to the stronger or faster man. But sooner or later, the man who wins is the man who thinks he can."

vi. Stop the Brain Drain: Limit Television Watching

Excessive television watching can adversely effect us in several ways:

1. It makes you less fit. People who watch television for less than one hour daily are fitter than those who watch for three to four hours daily.
2. It makes you obese. Two studies, one of 4,771 adult females (Tucker and Bagwell, 1991) and one of 6,138 males (Tucker and Friedman, 1989) have proven that television watching of three to four hours per day, doubled the risk of obesity in those persons compared to the persons who watched less than one hour of television per day. A recent study of 4,063 children, aged eight to 16, published in the Journal of American Medical Association (1998) concluded that excessive television watching by children made them fatter.
3. It makes you sedentary.
4. It makes you eat more, and it makes you eat more junk food.
5. It makes you mentally inactive during all the hours you watch television.

Reduce the damage television watching causes by limiting television watching to one hour or less per day, by not eating anything in front of the television, and by exercising—walking, lifting weights, doing jumping jacks or using the treadmill while watching television.

vii. Drink Alcohol: In Moderation

1. What is a drink and what is moderate drinking? A drink is defined as 12 oz of regular beer, 5 oz of wine or one and .5 oz of 80-proof distilled spirit. One or two drinks a day is moderate drinking.
2. How should you drink? Do not drink more than two drinks. Drink slowly. Do not mix alcohol with sedatives, tranquilizers or hypnotics. Do not mix different types of alcohol. If you use

spirits, drink with water, not sodas or juices, to cut down on sodium and calories.

3. Is alcohol a friend or a foe? Let us look at the friend. People who drink alcohol in moderation live longer than the people who do not drink at all. In 1996, the American Heart Association concluded that alcohol reduces mortality by stating, "the lowest mortality occurs in those who consume one or two drinks per day. In teetotalers or occasional drinkers, the mortality rates are higher than in those consuming one or two drinks per day" (AHA, 1996).

4. Moderate use of alcohol and exercise are the only two factors known to raise the level of "good" cholesterol (HDL). A recent Harvard Medical School study of 50,000 men showed that a glass of wine daily raises the level of HDL.

5. Alcohol reduces the tendency of blood to clot. Thus, it lowers the risk of heart attack from a clot in a coronary artery. A large number of recent studies have consistently demonstrated a reduction in coronary artery disease with moderate consumption of alcohol. There is a 30–50% reduction in the risk of developing coronary artery disease with consumption of one or two drinks of alcohol (AHA, 1996).

6. Another study in the New England Journal of Medicine (1997) also confirmed that overall death rates are lower among men and women consuming one alcoholic drink daily.

7. Alcohol in moderate amounts may also lower the risk of stroke caused by the blockage of arteries because it reduces the tendency of blood to clot (Sacco et al, 1999).

8. Moderate amounts of alcohol also improves digestion, reduces stress and promotes good sleep.

9. But, don't turn the friend into a foe! Protect your liver, don't binge. Also, more than two drinks increases the risk of cancer in general and breast cancer in particular. Avoid it in pregnancy. Finally, don't drink and drive.

10. The best prescription: Drink one glass of red wine daily.

viii. Use Seatbelts: On the Ground and in the Air

1. Seatbelts have been proven to be the most effective means of reducing fatalities and serious injuries in traffic accidents. The U.S. Department of Transportation reports that seatbelts save 9,500 lives per year.
2. There is one motor vehicle fatality every 12 minutes, one injury every 9 seconds and one crash every 5 seconds. Yet, only 66% of Americans use seatbelts.
3. Seatbelts and child safety seats prevent ejection, shift crash forces to the strongest parts of the body's structure, spread forces over a wide area of the body, allow the body to slow down gradually in a crash situation, protect the head and spinal cord.
4. Statistics show that increasing seatbelt use to 90% would prevent more than 5,000 fatalities, 132,000 injuries and save 8.8 billion dollars annually. Save your dollar, your body, your life.
5. Fight to enact stronger laws which would allot higher penalties for seatbelt and child safety seat rules not followed, enforce similar seatbelt laws and encourage public education.
6. Crusade for standard enforcement for seatbelt use.
7. Prevent drunken driving.
8. Child safety seats reduce the risk of fatal injury by 69% for infants younger than one year old and by 47% for toddlers one through four years old. Make sure you use them.
9. Do not assume that the presence of an airbag in your car obviates the need for a seatbelt. Airbags are not as protective as seatbelts. With or without airbags, use seatbelts.
10. If your rear seat has seatbelts, do not forget to wear them.

Our prescription: Click it in. Buckle up.

ix. Drive Defensively

Here are ten ways to arrive alive:

1. Be cautious, alert, courteous and responsible on the road.

2. Before you leave your driveway or parking spot, be sure each passenger is secured in the car, including children and pets.
3. Use a hands-free speakerphone. When using it, keep both hands on the wheel and both eyes on the road.
4. If you plan to drink, designate another driver. Follow the rules of the road, including not contesting the right of way or trying to race another car during a merge.
5. Notify the police if you see a car weaving, making wide turns, or stopping abruptly. The driver may be impaired.
6. Let impaired drivers pass you. If an oncoming car crosses towards you, pull over, sound the horn and flash your lights.
7. Driving too slowly can be as risky as speeding. Keep to the appropriate lanes, and drive with the flow of traffic.
8. At night, don't overdrive your headlights. Be sure you are not driving too fast to stop inside the illuminated area.
9. Maintain a safe following distance—approximately one second for every 10 miles of speed.
10. If you have car trouble, pull as far off the road as possible. Use flares and flashers, and stay off the roadway.

Our prescription: Drive safely to arrive alive.

x. Lobby Against Guns

Let us remind ourselves; a new handgun is produced every 20 seconds and is used to shoot someone every two minutes. At home, a gun is used during a domestic argument, a child gets killed accidentally and suicides are committed with guns all too often. Beyond the domestic scene, handguns are used each day in 33 rapes, 575 robberies and 1,116 assaults (American Civil Liberties Union, 1999). Handguns killed 40,000 people in the U.S. in 1993 and only 82 people in Japan, 76 people in Canada and 33 people in Great Britain the same year. We must realize that the gun is a significant menace. It was time to act a long time ago to ban guns. The lack of action reflects irresponsibility on our part. Guns shorten lives. This impacts against our mission to improve our lifespan.

X. Ten Simply Best Prescriptions

i. Be Optimistic

> *"Grow old along with me! The best is yet to be."*
>
> – Robert Browning

Do you see the glass as half empty or half full? That is the classic determination of whether you are an optimist or a pessimist. But there is much more to the definition.

No matter how it develops, pessimism can be hazardous to health. It snatches the drive out of us, makes us less productive and affects our defense systems by weakening the immune system. Optimism is a powerful builder of the body, mind and spirit, and hence a nurturer of good health.

Now, concerning optimism, we cannot change our childhood, but we can change our attitudes. Here are ten steps to being more optimistic suggested by Coleman and Gurin (1993):

1. Think about your attitudes in the area in which you would like to be more optimistic.
2. Consider if these attitudes are realistic.
3. Set small, immediate goals for changing your attitudes.
4. Each time you reach those goals, reward yourself.
5. Make a point to spend time with people who are optimistic.
6. Learn to laugh and be playful about your quest for optimism.
7. Remind yourself that optimism leads to action.
8. Enlist the support of family and friends.
9. Improve your lifestyle based on an attitude of optimism.
10. Use these suggestions however they serve you best. If you have some setbacks, don't blame yourself. Habits die hard.

Acting on these tips will make you confident and happier and healthier. They're sure to make life more worth living and inspire you to enjoy it for a long, long time.

ii. Stay Mentally Active: Always be A Busy Bee

Here are some ways to exercise your brain, whatever your age:

1. Go back to school.
2. Join a club.
3. Volunteer. Tutor a schoolchild or an adult.
4. Share your experience.
5. Watch mentally stimulating television programs such as *Jeopardy*, or *Wheel of Fortune*.
6. Use the Internet.
7. Stay in touch with current events, friends, and information about health, and investments.
8. Manage your money. Stay mentally active by studying investments, and consulting with brokers.
9. Take a part-time job.
10. Do an art project or learn a musical instrument.

At any age, staying active is a major component of good mental and physical health. It becomes more important as one grows older. You can be busy at home too. Do little things like playing with children, cleaning the house, washing a car or watering plants. If you are looking for something away from home here are some suggestions:

1. Look out for listings of community events.
2. Get involved at your temple, church or other institution.
3. Find a place to volunteer such as a school, hospital.
4. Spend time with a child, be it with your own grandchild.
5. Take up a hobby.
6. Exercise!
7. Get a part-time job.
8. Spend time in a book store or library. Read, write, or simply surf around on the Internet.
9. Find an organization that interests you, and join it! Get involved.
10. Don't forget your friends. Simply spending quiet time playing games or discussing events can be enough to keep busy and going to the century mark!

Our prescription: An active body means an active mind. There are a lot of ways to keep busy. Find the ones you like, and stick to them.

iii. Learn The Latest Things

Your foremost source for information regarding new research and advancements that could affect your health should be your doctor and the medical organizations. Here are some other ways to keep up with the latest findings.

1. Read the latest books and articles in magazines.
2. Subscribe to an online mailing list through one of the Internet sites.
3. Stay tuned to your television for health-related programs.
4. Take classes at your local college or university
5. Talk to your doctor, clergy, friend, relative or teacher. Keep an open mind, stay informed about new things.

iv. Be Disciplined

Achieving a goal takes a lot of hard work and hard work takes liberal doses of dedication and discipline. There is so much that goes along with living to be 100. You have to eat right, exercise, keep a positive attitude, and do other things such as quitting smoking, losing weight. To accomplish all these things takes unflinching discipline. Here are a few tips to help you on your way:

1. Remember why you set the goal in the first place.
2. If you feel unmotivated or weak, ask yourself this question, "How will this help me live to be 100?" If you can't answer that question with something positive, then think again about lapsing into bad habits.
3. Call a friend to talk.
4. Read a book or a magazine.
5. Run an errand, clean your house, or find other chores to keep yourself busy.
6. Remind yourself how much better you'll feel once goals have been accomplished that you've set out to do.

7. Make a list of reasons why you should stick to your goal, and read them when feeling unmotivated.
8. Take a walk around the neighborhood to clear your head.
9. Relax. Don't be too hard on yourself if you slip. Sometimes, small indulgences can keep us sane, so long as they don't get out of control.
10. By being disciplined, you can slowly turn a bad habit into something good. Discipline yourself to achieve your goals.

v. Eat Right

We started with COMMANDMENT I, *Thou shalt eat healthy*. Eating right is the most important factor in maintaining good health. We've learned that eating the wrong foods endangers you with a host of medical conditions.

Refer back to the chapters which tell you what good foods are. You know about the "famous" diets, what to eat at formal restaurants and at fast food places. All that remains for you to do is use all the information in this book and eat right.

vi. Exercise Regularly: The Perfect Panacea

We hear it all the time on television, in magazines and in newspapers: exercise and feel better. You know that exercising can help you live a longer life and help stem your body's physical decline. A small increase in physical activity, such as walking, yields many benefits including reduction in the risk of debilitating diseases such as coronary artery disease.

Exercise is a way to make sure your body is working at its peak levels, and to help ensure that you do what you can to make your health and your goal of living to be 100 attainable. Plus, exercise is a great way to clear your mind, relax you and help you feel better. So why not get up and do something for yourself that will not only improve the way you look and keep your body healthy, but can also improve your mind and your attitude?

Start right, go slow, build up to more intense levels, be regular. When you exercise, it's very important to remember to stretch, warm up and cool down after every activity. It minimizes soreness and helps your body get adjusted to the physical activity.

Finding an activity is easy. Some tips for healthy aerobic activity: Walk or run. Swim or ride a bike. Join fitness and health education classes. Try ballroom dancing. Run your errands. Take your pet outside. Take your grandchild to the park! Push your grandson on a swing, push your granddaughter in her stroller, just make sure you're not sitting on a park bench, watching them run around.

vii. Don't Smoke: Butt Out To Breathe Better

Is there anyone still smoking? If you are, please note: one in every five deaths in the U.S. is related to smoking. Ten million Americans have lost their lives due to cigarette smoking since 1964. Look back to the chapter on smoking to remind you about the statistical score. Even though cigarette smoking causes more preventable deaths from cardiovascular disease and cancer than any other modifiable risk factor, most smokers do not view themselves at increased risk of heart disease or cancer (Ayanian, Cleary, 1999). If you are one of them follow the tips in the chapter on smoking.

In the final analysis we believe there is no better and more polite way to write a prescription than to say, "Thank you for not smoking."

viii. Get Enough Sleep: The Best Energizer

Remember this short list of actions to get good sleep:

1. Form good habits: go to bed at a regular time and get up the same time every morning. Make sure your bedroom is dark and your bed and room temperature comfortable. Spend the most lavishly on a good mattress. You spend many hours on it.
2. Read a book, turn the television off.
3. Drink a glass of warm skim milk.

4. Axe alcohol, nix nicotine, avoid coffee, tea and caffeinated sodas for six to eight hours before going to bed. Avoid refined carbohydrates.
5. Use sleeping medications only as prescribed by your physician. Avoid using them for extended periods. Avoid them completely if you can.
6. Take a warm bath before going to bed.
7. Avoid long naps during the daytime.
8. Don't fight sleep. Don't toss and turn. Leave the bed and walk around if you can't fall asleep.

Our prescription: If you sleep well, you will function better and live longer.

viii. Recognize the "Rights": Preserve Your Mind-Body Connection

This is the best connection you will make in life. As we age, it is easy to feel a sense of helplessness, that life is swirling out of control, that we cannot handle ourselves as well as we once could. There is something that we can do which can have an effect on how we think. That is, maintaining a positive outlook and not "losing it". This could mean the difference between a good life and a bad life.

Depression is the biggest breaker of the mind-body connection. Treat it. Somewhere between 12–20% of the nation's elderly population (people over age 70) show some signs of depression. With that, there is a drop in physical abilities (Penninx, 1998).

Stay active. Remain positive and upbeat. Maintain a positive connection between your mind and your body.

Correct the problems that may affect the strength of the mind-body connection. Wipe out stress. Address your emotional problems. Find friends and cultivate relationships. Seek peace. Stop abusing your body with bad foods, a sedentary life and excesses of alcohol and drugs. Preserve and protect your body and your mind, and your spirits will rise to make things right.

ix. Just Do It

"Success is the prize to be won. Action is the road to it."

– O. Henry

"As soon as you feel too old to do a thing, do it."

– Margaret Deland

The time for action is now. It is never too early. It is never too late. Each of the above 99 prescriptions will increase longevity. Exercise, eat right and stay trim. Be disciplined and determined. Remain optimistic and resilient. Stay creative mentally and physically. Stop smoking and abusing alcohol and drugs. Relax, pray, love, and laugh. Learn, help others, and be involved. Celebrate each day. Think young and work to be 100.

Our prescription: No excuses, start today. The best prescription of all is: Just do It!

x. Promise Yourself A 100th Birthday

Being 100 is not a sin or a crime. At the turn of the 20th century, the thought of living to 100 would have been unimaginable. Back then, people hardly lived to see their 50th birthdays, let alone their 100th. Nowadays, at the start of the third millennium, each morning a new centenarian is celebrated on NBC's *Today* show. That's quite a change from almost 100 years ago.

The human mind can be a powerful thing. A person's will power can topple any obstacles once the mind is set to do something. So why not be stubborn about living to your 100th birthday?

It's not an easy task, but with a little work and determination, anything is possible. With a goal clearly set in mind, a positive attitude, willpower and courage can take you to the century mark.

In this book, we have provided a number of prescriptions for making it to 100. Using these as a guide, you can incorporate the steps into your life and make them your lifestyle. Some are easy pills to swallow, others are not, but living to be 100 doesn't come without a little work. Just find what works for you, and do it!

Throughout the book every factor that can promote health and improve your life span is discussed. A major emphasis has been placed on nutrition, exercise, weight control, and smoking cessation which can lead to prevention of heart and blood vessel disease. The subjects of prevention of heart disease, cancer, accidents, immune disease, infectious diseases that cut your life short or can disable you are addressed. You are also handed powerful tools to reduce stress through praying, meditation, love and laughter. There are longevity pearls everywhere in the book.

As provided at the outset, we have remained committed to presenting sound advice based on sound medical principles. No gimmicks, no quackery, no misleading information. Be assured it is safe to follow.

Now that you have read the book it is time to digest the contents. This is what Francis Bacon said, "Some books are to be tasted, others to be swallowed, and some few to be chewed and digested." Take this book and run to get to the goal line.

In sum, here are ten ways you can fulfill your promise to living to 100 years of age:

1. Watch what you eat.
2. Exercise your body.
3. Exercise your mind.
4. Stay involved with something, anything, all your life.
5. Adopt a positive mental attitude.
6. Don't let your age limit you.
7. Surround yourself with happy, positive people of all ages.
8. Get in touch with your spiritual side.
9. Stay closely involved with your family.
10. Bring your body, mind, and the spirit together to create a formula to live to be 100 or longer, and healthier.

References

Albom, M. (1997). *Tuesdays with Morrie.* New York, NY: Doubleday.

Alcohol consumption and mortality among middle-aged and elderly U.S. adults. (1997). *New England Journal of Medicine, 337*, 1705-1714.

American Association of Retired Persons. (1987). Activities with Impact. [pamphlet]. Washington, DC, 13.

American Cancer Society. (1997). Website: www.cancer.org.

American Civil Liberties Union. (1999). Gun stats. Website: http://www.aclu-Sc.org/GunStats.htm.

American Dietetic Association. (1998). Ten great ways to fiber up. Web site: http://www.eatright.org.

American Heart Association. (1997). Guide to primary prevention of cardiovascular diseases. Website: http://www.amhrt.org/scientific/statements/1997/059701.html.

American Heart Association. (1996). Website: http://www.amhrt.org.

Anderson, G. (1995). *The 22 Non-Negotiable Laws of Wellness.* San Francisco, Ca: Harper San Francisco, 169, 175, 176.

Anderson, R.E., et al. (1998). Relationship of physical activity and television watching with body weight and level of fatness. *Journal of the American Medical Association, 279*, 938-42.

Appel, L.J., Espeland, M.A., Wheaton, P.K., et al. (1998). Sodium reduction and weight loss in the treatment of hypertension in older persons. *Journal of the American Medical Association, 279*, 839-840.

Ayanian, J.Z and Cleary, P.D. (1999). Perceived risks of heart disease and cancer among cigarette smokers. *Journal of the American Medical Association, 281*, 1019-1021.

Batmanghelidj, F. (1997). *Your Body's Many Cries for Water.* Falls Church, VA: Global Health Solutions, Inc.

Bradshaw, J. (1992). *Creating Love.* New York, NY: Bantam, 311.

Braunwald, Fauci, Isselbacher, Kasper, Martin, Wilson, Eds. (1994). *Harrison's Principles of Internal Medicine,* (13th edition). New York, NY: McGraw Hill, Inc.

Brody, J. (1997). *The New York Times Book of Health.* NY, NY: Times Books.

Burns, G. (1983). *How to Live to be 100—or More. The Ultimate Diet, Sex and Exercise Book.* New York, NY: G.P. Putnam's Sons.

Buscaglia, L. (1992). *Born for Love.* New York, NY: Fawcett Columbine.

Byrd R. (1988). University of California at San Francisco.

Carper, J. (1995). *Stop Aging Now.* New York, NY: Harper Collins Publisher.

Coleman, D. and Gurin, J. (1993). *Mind/Body Medicine.* Yonkers, NY: Consumer Reports Books, 364.

Dossey L. (1996). *Prayer in Good Medicine.* San Francisco, CA: Harper.

Dyer, W. (1999, March 18). *"How to Get What you Really, Really, Really, Really Want."* WLRN-TV.

Dyer, W. (1995). *Your Sacred Self.* New York, NY: Harper Collins.

Fatteh, A. with Fatteh, N. (1999). *At Journey's End: A Complete Guide to Funerals and Funeral Planning.* Los Angeles, CA: Health Information Press.

Gonzalez-Balado J.L. (1996). *Mother Theresa, In My Own Words.* New York, NY: Random House.

Hite, S. (1981). *The Hite Report on Male Sexuality.* New York, NY: Ballantine.

Hope, R.E. (1998). *Greater Late Than Never. Fulfilling Your Dreams After 50.* Atlanta, GA: Longstreet.

International Center for Humor and Health. (1999, February 26). Website: www.humorandhealth.com.

Johns Hopkins Family Health Book. (1999). New York, NY: Harper Collins.

Johnson, D.W. (1998). *Feel 30 for the Next 50 Years.* New York, NY: Avon Books.

Johnson, J. and Klein, L. (1994). *I Can Cope. Staying Healthy with Cancer.* Minneapolis, MN: Chronimed Publishing.

Lazarou, J., et al. (1998). Incidence of adverse drug reactions in hospitalized patients. *Journal of the American Medical Association, 279*, 1200-1205.

Klag, M..J. et al. (1999). *Johns Hopkins Family Health Book.* New York, NY: Harper Collins Publishers.

Matthews, D.A., Larson, D.B. and Barry, C.P. (1994). *The Faith Factor: An Annotated Bibliography of Clinical Research on Spiritual Subjects.* John Templeton Foundation.

Myers, D.G. (2000) Psychology (6th ed.). New York, NY: Worth Publishers. (www.davidmyers.org, Chapter 17.)

Natow, A.B. and Heslin, J. (1999). *The Most Complete Food Counter.* New York, NY: Pocket Books, Division of Simon and Schuster.

Orenstrin, R. and Sobel, S. (1996). *The Healthy Mind Healthy Body.* New York, NY: Time Warner, 33-34.

Ornish D, et al. (1998). Intensive lifestyle changes for reversal of coronary heart disease. *Journal of the American Medical Association, 280*, 2001-7.

Ornish D. (1991). *Reversing Heart Disease.* New York, NY: Ballantine Books.

Patient page: Weight management. (1999). *Journal of the American Medical Association, 281(3)*, 296.

Penninx, B. et al. (1998). Depressive Symptoms and Physical Decline in Community Dwelling Persons. *Journal of the American Medical Association, 279*, 1720-1726.

Peterson, W. (1997). *The Art of Living.* New York, NY: Bristol Parks Books, 146.

Physicians Desk Reference for Nonprescription Drugs. (1998). Montvale, NJ: Medical Economics Co., Inc.

Pratt M. (1999). Benefits of lifestyle activity vs. structured exercise, editorial. *Journal of the American Medical Association, 281(4),* 375.

Rendell, et al. (1999). Sildenafil for treatment of erectile dysfunction in men with diabetes. *Journal of the American Medical Association, 281,* 421.

Ricco, D. (1998). *Superfoods for Life.* East Rutherford, NJ: Berkley Publishing.

Rinzler, C.A. (1997). *Nutrition for Dummies.* Foster City, CA: IDG Books Worldwide, Inc., p 35.

Sacco, et al. (1999). The protective effect of alcohol consumption on ischemic stroke. *Journal of the American Medical Association, 281,* 53-60.

Smith, M.H. and Smith, S. (1999). *The Retirement Source Book.* Los Angeles, CA: Lowell House.

Stevens, P. *Beating Job Burnout.* (1995). Chicago, IL: NTC Publishing, 25-27.

Tucker, L.A. and Bagwell, M. (1991, July). Television viewing and obesity in adult females. *American Journal of Public Health, 81(7),* 908-11.

Tucker, L.A. and Friedman, G.M. (1989, April). Television viewing and obesity in adult males. *American Journal of Public Health, 79(4),* 516-518.

United States Department of Agriculture. (1998). Website. http://www.os.dhhs.gov.

Appendix A

TABLE A.1
Recommended Childhood Immunization Schedule
United States, January - December 1998

	Hepatitis B		Diptheria/Tetanus Toxoids/Pertussis	Haemophilus influenza type B	Poliovirus	Measles-Mumps-Rubella	Varicella Virus
Birth	Hep B-1						
1 mo		Hep B-2					
2 mos			DTaP or DTP	Hib	Polio		
4 mos			DTaP or DTP	Hib	Polio		
6 mos	Hep B-3		DTaP or DTP	Hib	Polio		
12 mos				Hib	Polio	MMR	Var
15 mos			DTaP or DTP				
18 mos							
4-6 yrs			DTaP or DTP		Polio	MMR	
11-12 yrs	Hep B-3		Td			MMR	Var
14-16 yrs							

KEY: Range of Acceptable Ages for Vaccine | Vaccines to be Assessed and Administered if Necessary

TABLE A.2
Body Mass Index (BMI)*

Weight (lb)	4'10"	5'0"	5'2"	5'4"	5'6"	5'8"	5'10"	6'0"	6'2"
125	26	24	23	22	20	19	18	17	16
130	27	25	24	22	21	20	19	18	17
135	28	26	25	23	22	21	19	18	17
140	29	27	26	24	23	21	20	19	18
145	30	28	27	25	23	22	21	20	19
150	31	29	27	26	24	23	22	20	19
155	32	30	28	27	25	24	22	21	20
160	34	31	29	28	26	24	23	22	21
165	35	32	30	28	27	25	24	22	21
170	36	33	31	29	28	26	24	23	22
175	37	34	32	30	28	27	25	24	23
180	38	35	33	31	29	27	26	25	23
185	39	36	34	32	30	28	27	25	24
190	40	37	35	33	31	29	27	26	24
195	41	38	36	34	32	30	28	27	25
200	42	39	37	34	32	30	29	27	26
205	43	40	38	35	33	31	29	28	26
210	44	41	38	36	34	32	30	29	27
215	45	42	39	37	35	33	31	29	28
220	46	43	40	38	36	34	32	30	28
225	47	44	41	39	36	34	32	31	29
230	48	45	42	40	37	35	33	31	30

Height (ft, in)

BMI values that correlate to a higher risk of adverse effects on health:

BMI = 30 kg/m²

BMI = 27 kg/m² in the presence of risk factors

*BMI is defined as body weight (in kg) divided by height (in m²)

Appendix B

TABLE B.1
Vitamins: Symptoms And Signs Of Deficiency And Overdose

Vitamin	Male RDA	Female RDA	Deficiency	Overdose
Vitamin A	1000 mcg	800 mcg	Night blindness, dry skin, weight loss, poor bone growth, diarrhea, acne, insomnia, fatigue	Bleeding from gums or mouth sores, confusion, diarrhea, double vision, dry skin, hair loss, skin peeling, increased liver/spleen size
Vitamin D	5 mcg	5 mcg	Rickets (childhood disease with malformation of bones and joints), late tooth development, osteomalacia (adults, pain in bones, easily broken bones)	High blood pressure, irregular heartbeat, weight loss, seizures, physical growth retardation, premature hardening of arteries
Vitamin E	10 mg	8 mg	Irritable, edema, hemolytic anemia, lethargy, nerve dysfunction	High doses deplete vitamin A, (signs of vitamin A deficiency)
Vitamin C (Ascorbic Acid)	60 mg	60 mg	Scurvy (muscle weakness, swollen gums, depression), easy bruising, nosebleeds, anemia, frequent infections, slow wound healing	Flushed face, headache, abdominal cramps, diarrhea, nausea, vomiting

TABLE B.1 continued

Vitamin	Male RDA	Female RDA	Deficiency	Overdose
Thiamin (Vitamin B1)	1.1 mg	1.5 mg	Loss of appetite, fatigue, nausea, depression, memory loss, Wernicke's encephalopathy, decrease reflexes, tender or atrophy of muscles	Hypertensive reactions, drowsiness
Riboflavin (Vitamin B2)	1.3 mg	1.7 mg	Cracks and sores of mouth, lip/tongue inflammation, sensitivity to light by eyes, insomnia, itching of skin	Unlikely to cause toxicity unless renal failure
Niacin (Vitamin B3)	15 mg	19 mg	Delirium, fatigue, swollen or red tongue, scaly skin, diarrhea, dermatitis	Body flush, nausea, weakness, diarrhea, high blood sugar
Vitamin B6 (Pyridoxine)	1.6 mg	2.0 mg	Weakness, confusion, irritable, nervous, insomnia, poor coordination, anemia, muscle twitching	Nerve damage, kidney stone formation
Folate (Folic Acid)	180 mcg	200 mcg	Megalobastic anemia (large and uneven sized red blood cells), weak, irritable, lack of energy and appetite, confusion, diarrhea	Kidney stones, appetite loss, flatulence
Vitamin B12	2 mcg	2 mcg	Profound fatigue, nerve damage, weakness, confusion, nausea, poor memory	If taken with Vitamin C can cause nosebleed

TABLE B.2

Minerals: Symptoms And Signs Of Deficiency And Overdose

Mineral	Male RDA	Female RDA	Deficiency	Overdose
Calcium	800-1200 mg	800-1200 mg	Osteoperosis, osteomalacia (fractures, muscle cramps), children - increased cavities, stunted growth, high blood pressure	Confusion, slow or irregular heartbeat, bone or muscle pain, nausea or vomiting
Phosphorous	800-1200 mg	800-1200 mg	Fragile bones, weakness, poor appetite	Seizure, irregular heartbeat, shortness of breath
Magnesium	350 mg	280 mg	Muscle weakness, cramps, tremors, confusion, memory loss, hallucinations, irregular heartbeat	Nausea, vomiting, low blood pressure, muscle weakness, heartbeat irregularity
Iron	10 mg	15 mg	Fatigue, anemia, pale appearance of skin, mucus membranes, heart palpitations with exertion	Diarrhea, bloody vomit or stools, weakness, convulsions, coma
Zinc	15 mg	12 mg	Loss of appetite, decreased ability to taste food, poor wound healing, male infertility, glossitis, stomatitis	Effects on kidney, liver or spleen function
Iodine	150 mcg	150 mcg	Goiter (swollen thyroid gland) mental and physical retardation, sluggish behavior	Confusion, irregular heartbeat, difficulty breathing, black or tarry stool

TABLE B.2 *continued*

Mineral	Male RDA	Female RDA	Deficiency	Overdose
Selenium	70 mcg	55 mcg	Muscle pain, weakness of heart	Nausea, vomiting, muscle ache, abdominal pain, anemia
Copper	2 mg	2 mg	Anemia, low white blood cell count causing increased susceptibility to infection; poor collagen formation, hair loss	Delusions, insomnia, hallucinations
Manganese	2-5 mg	2-5 mg	No known effects in humans	No known effects in humans
Chromium	50-200 mcg	50-200 mcg	Numbness of extremities, disturbance of fat, glucose, protein metabolism	Low toxicity, skin, liver, kidney

Index

Accidents, 259
Action plans, ten decades, 249
Ads, 272
Alcohol
    calories in, 291
    drinking, 341
Aging, 5
AIDS
    virus, 258
    prevention, 283
American Cancer Society, 277
American Cancer Society diet, 47
American Diabetic Association, 277
American Dietetic Association, 277
American Heart Association, 47, 277
American Lung Association, 277
American Medical Association, 277
American Restaurant, 63
American Steakhouse, 62
Amino Acids in beans, 36
Anger, control of, 305
Antioxidants, 103
Arby's, 82
Arts, 307
Attitude, positive, 340

Beans, 36
Be a loser, 313
Be disciplined, 347
Be generous, 325
Be optimistic, 345
Be resilient, 337
Behavior modification, 315
Beliefs, 5
Believe in yourself, 339
Beta carotene, 104
Bicycling, 164
    basic principles, 168
    benefits of, 168
    elements of preparation, 165
    fitness for, 165
    goals, 169
    helmet, shoes, clothing for, 166
    nutrition, hydration for, 166
    risks of, 168
    safety factors, 167
    stretching for, 165
    training for, 165
Birthday, 100th, 351
Bland diet, 99
BMI Table, 358
BMI (Body Mass Index) 198, 201
Body abusing, 277
Body parts, 227
Brain, 271
Brain-body poisons, 272
Brain drain, 341
Breakfast, 288
Breathe right, 285
Burger King, 77
Burnout, 338

Caffeine content in beverages, 217
Calcium, 114
    best sources, 115
    daily requirement, 116
    high calcium diet, 98
Calorie counts, 313
    in alcohol, 291
    in soda, 317
Cancer, 260
    anti-cancer diet, 89
    prevention protocols, 284
Carbohydrates, 27
    complex, 27
    refined, 27
Cardiovascular system, 238
    protective steps, 239
Caring for your body, 271
CDC (Centers for Disease Control), 277
Celebrate each day, 336
Change career, 275
Check-ups, 278

Chelation therapy, 126
Chinese restaurant, 63
Cholesterol, 29
    bad, 30
    good, 30
    HDL, 30
    in foods, 30
    LDL, 28, 30
    total, 28, 30
    VLDL, 30
Chronic conditions, common, 229
Chylomicrons, 30
Coenzyme Q^{10}, 134
Commandments, 11
    Commandment I, 25
    good sleep, 217
    health, 11
Compliance with medical advice, 278
Connection, mind-body, 350
Constipation, 240, 274
Contentment, 310
Control anger, 305
Cool down, 299
Coping, 338
Crusade, anti-smoking, 196

Dairy Queen, 81
Dance, 326
Death, causes of, 228
Decades of life, causes of death, 249
Depression, 273
Dermatologic system, 235
    tips to preserve, 236
Develop self-respect, 339
DHEA, 127
Diabetes diet, 87
Diet
    anti-cancer, 86
    calcium, high, 98
    diabetic, 87
    gout, 92
    healthy individual, 83
    heart-healthy, 85
    high fiber, 96
    hypoglycemia, 89
    low salt, 94
    medicinal, 83
    ulcer, 99
Diet pills, 204, 318
    side effects of, 205
Diet prescriptions, 287
Diet regimens, prescribed, 294
Diets, ten famous, 42
    American Cancer Society, 49
    Dean Ornish, 48
    Food Pyramid, 43
    Jenny Craig, 52
    Nutri/System, 56
    Pritikin, 49
    Scarsdale, 50
    Slim Fast, 53
    Step I and Step II, 45
    Weight Watcher's, 54
Discipline, 347
Do it, 351
Domino's, 80
Don't retire, 275
Don't smoke, 349
Drink alcohol, 341
Drive defensively, 343

Eat
    heart healthy, 85, 290
    right ways, 287, 348
Endocrine system, 233
Endorphins, 247
EKG (electrocardiogram) 18
Emergency medicines, 282
EPA (Environmental Protection
    Agency), 277
Essential amino acids, 36
Exercises, 145
    benefits, 146
    burnout, 147
    energy expenditure, 146
    excuses for not exercising, 295
    in water, 301
    safe, 297

Index

ten best, 145
Exercise, without exercising, 296
    basic requirements, 300
    for weight loss, 314
    right place, 298
Fads, 272
Falls, prevention, 286
Family history, 280
Fast foods, 74
    Arby's, 82
    Burger King, 77
    Dairy Queen, 81
    Domino's, 80
    Hardee's, 79
    Kentucky Fried Chicken, 78
    McDonald's, 76
    Pizza Hut, 78
    Taco Bell, 81
    Wendy's, 79
Fat, 28
Fat, saturated, intake, 46
Feelings, 324
Fiber, 293
    high fiber diet, 96
    sources, 98
Folate, 116
    best sources of, 118
    daily requirement, 118
Food
    as medicine, 83
    Food Pyramid, 30, 33, 43, 288
    for longevity, 25
Free radicals, 103, 290
French restaurant, 70
Friends, 323
Fruits, 30
    ten best, 32
Fundamental beliefs, 5

Garlic, 138
Gastrointestinal system, 239
    tips to protect, 240
Genesis 6:3, 9
Ginger, 137

Gingko, 136
Ginseng, 134
Glutathione, 133
Goal of this book, 9
Gold standards, 13
Gout, anti-gout diet, 92
Grains, 33
    ten best sources, 35
Group activities, 324
Growth hormone, 131
Guiness Book of World Records, 6, 7
Guns, lobby against, 344

Hardee's, 79
HDL (High Density Cholesterol), 30
Health organization, 276
Healthy individual diet, 85
Heart disease, 257
Heart healthy diet, 85
Help, volunteer, 325
Hematologic system, 231
    ways to protect, 232
HGH (Human Growth Hormone), 131
Hobbies, 307
Hypertension, 263
Hypoglycemia diet, 89

Immune system, 245
Immunization schedule, childhood, 357
Immunize children, 285
Independence, personal, 331
Indian restaurant, 71
Influenza, 265
Insomnia
    causes of, 216
    dangers of, 215
    medical causes of, 220
International restaurants, 59
Introduction, 5
Iron, best sources, 232
Italian restaurant, 65

Japanese restaurant, 69
Jenny Craig diet, 52

Just do it, 351

Kentucky Fried Chicken, 78
Killers, major, 257

Laughter, 303
LDL (Low Density Cholesterol), 28, 30
Learn latest things, 347
Let go, 306
Life expectancies, 7, 8
Lipoproteins, 30
Lobby against guns, 344
Loneliness, 320
Loner, 320
Longevity in a pill box, 279
Love, 222, 335
    essential elements of, 222
    healing power, 222
    longevity, 224
    spousal, 223
Loved ones, 321

Magic bullets, 103
Major killers, 257
Marriage, 322
McDonald's, 76
Medical check-ups, 278
Medical prescriptions, 278
Medicines, emergency, 282
Medicine, priceless, 303
Meditate, 333
Melatonin, 129
Menus
    anti-cancer, 86
    bland diet, 99
    calcium, high, 98
    diabetic, 87
    gout, 92
    healthy individual, 83
    heart-healthy, 85
    high fiber, 96
    hypoglycemia, 89
    low salt, 94
Mexican restaurant, 68

Middle Eastern restaurant, 66
Mind, expand, 328
Minerals, best sources, 121
    deficiency, 361
Milk, low fat, 292
Murder, 265
Musculoskeletal system, 244

Nervous system, 227
    ways to protect, 230
Nice thing, say daily, 330
Nutri/system Weight Loss Program, 56
Nutritional value, common drinks, 95

Obesity, 202, 262
    correction of cause, 312
    prevention, 311
    treatment options, 203
objectives of the book, 6
oils, good and bad, 29
Olympics, senior, 324
optimism, 345
organizations, health, 276
Ornish, Dean Program, 48
OTC (Over the Counter) Drugs, 279, 281

Pamper yourself, 303
Panacea, perfect, 348
Peace, 335
People person, 320
Personal independence, 331
Pill box, 279
Pills, diet, 318
Pizza Hut, 78
Pneumonia, vaccinate, 265
Poisons, 272
Positive attitude, 340
Pray, 332
Prescriptions, 271
    diet, 287
    exercise, 295
    formula for, 17
    general, 338
    longevity, 13

Index

medical, 278
mental, spiritual, 329
one hundred, 271
primary, 11
reducing stress, 303
simply best, 345
social emotional, 320
weight control, 311
Priceless medicine, 303
Pritikin diet, 49
Promise, 351
Protein, 25
daily requirement, 26
Protocols, cancer prevention, 284
PSA (Prostatic Specific Antigen), 18
Pyramid, Food, 43, 44, 288

Quacks, 272
Question, Big, 6

RDA (Recommended Daily Allowance), 112
Recognize the "rights", 350
Relationship, 322
Resilience, 337
Respiratory system, 236
ways to protect, 237
Restaurants, 59
American, 63
Chinese, 61
French, 70
Great American Steakhouse, 62
Indian, 71
International, 59
Italian, 65
Japanese, 69
Mexican, 68
Middle Eastern, 66
Seafood Gourmet, 64
Thai, 72
Retire, don't, 275
Right ways to eat, 287
Running, 162
right ways of running, 163
tips for novice runner, 163

Safe exercises, 297
Safe sex, 327
Salt, 37
low-salt diet, 94
Saturated fat intake, 46
Scarsdale Diet, 50
Schedule, immunization, 357
Seafood restaurant, 64
Seatbelts, 343
Self respect, 339
Sex, 308
Sleep, 214, 349
amount needed, 214
benefits of good sleep, 216
commandments for sleep, 217
insomnia, 215
shift work and, 219
sleep levels, necessary, 215
Slim Fast Diet, 53
Smoking, 193, 349
secondhand smoke, 195
smokeless tobacco, 196
ten steps to stop, 194
Snack sensibly, 316
Soda, calories in, 317
Soft drinks, 317
Soy, 39
Stay mentally active, 346
Steakhouse, 62
Step I and Step II Diets, 45
Storytellers, 13
Stress, 207
acute, 211
banishment of, 210
busting strategies, 211
creation of, 210
domestic, 207
effect on health, 209
external/ environmental, 207
job, 209
level, major life events, 208
positive and negative, 209

prescriptions to reduce, 303
Stressors, 309
Stretch
    yawn, 148
    here and there, 299
Stretching, 148
    benefits of, 149
    calf, 152
    chest, 152
    diagrams, 155
    extremities, 152
    for executives, 151
    front leg, 153
    groin, 154
    hamstring, 153
    in bed, 150
    in water, 178
    jumping jacks, 151
    legs and buttocks, 153
    lower back, 154
    principles of, 149
    shoulder, 152
    shoulder and chest, 153
    side, 152
    sit-up, 154
    thigh and hip muscles, 153
    trunk rotation, 152
    when to, 150
    where to, 150
Stroke, 228
Suicides, 264
Sunset years, 275
Supplements, vitamin and mineral, 112
Swim, 301
System, 227
    cardiovascular, 230
    dermatologic, 235
    endocrine, 233
    gastrointestinal, 239
    hematologic, 231
    immune, 245
    musculoskeletal, 244
    nervous, 227
    respiratory, 236
    urinary, 242
Taco Bell, 81
Television, watching, 341
Thai restaurant, 72
Travel, 328

Ulcer diet, 99
Unexpected events, 304
Urinary system, 242
    ways to prevent disease, 243

Vaccinate, 265
Vegetables, 33
    ten best, 34
Vitamin A, 104
    best sources of, 105
    deficiency and overdose, 104
Vitamin B12, 120
    best sources of, 122
    deficiency, consequences of, 120
Vitamin C, 106
    best sources of, 106
    deficiency and overdose, 107
Vitamin D, 113
    deficiency and overdose, 113
Vitamin E, 107
    best sources of, 109
    deficiency and overdose, 108
Vitamins and minerals, 290
Vitamins, deficiency signs and
    symptoms, 359
Volunteering, 325

Walking, 158, 301
    benefits, 158
    guidelines for seniors, 160
    right ways to walk, 159
    safety tips, 160
Warm up, 299
Water, 38, 294
Water Exercises, 171, 301
    aerobic exercises, 178
    benefits of, 171
    diagrams, 184

stretching exercises, 174
Weight control, 198
    desired weight, calorie maintenance table, 199
Weight management, 202
    behavior modification, 203
    commitment and compliance, 202
    exercise, 203
    sensible eating, 203
    special considerations, 203
Weight, optimum, 312
Weight Watcher's Diet, 54
Wendy's, 79
WHO (World Health Organization), 277
Will to enjoy life, 329

Xenical, 204

Yawn stretch, 148
Young, associate with, 329
Young, think, 329
Yo-Yo, 318

Zinc, 117
    best sources of, 120